CHINESE MEDICAL CHARACTERS
VOLUME ONE: BASIC VOCABULARY
中医用字
第一册：基本词汇辑

Zhōng Yī Yòng Zì Dì Yì Cè: Jī Běn Cí Huì Jí

Chinese Medicine Language Series

Nigel Wiseman 魏迺杰

Yǔhuán Zhāng 张宇环

Edited by Michael Helme

Paradigm Publications
Taos New Mexico USA

Chinese Medical Characters
Volume One: Basic Vocabulary
中医用字第一册：基本词汇辑
Zhōng Yī Yòng Zì Dì Yī Cè: Jī Běn Cí Huì Jí
Chinese Medicine Language Series
Nigel Wiseman and ZhāngYǔhuán
Copyright © 2003 Paradigm Publications

Library of Congress Cataloging-in-Publication Data

Wiseman, Nigel.
  Chinese medical characters / Nigel Wiseman, Yéuhâuan Zhåang ; edited
by Michael Helme = Zhong yi yong zi / Wei Naijie, Zhåang Yéuhâuan.
      p. ; cm. -- (Chinese medicine language series)
Includes bibliographical references and index.
Text in English and Chinese, including Pinyin.
   ISBN 0-912111-68-2 (pbk. : vol. 1 : alk. paper)
  1.   Medicine, Chinese--Terminology.
   [DNLM: 1.   Medicine, Chinese Traditional--Terminology--Chinese. 2.
Medicine, Chinese Traditional--Terminology--English.   WB 15 W814c
2003] I. Title: Zhong yi yong zi. II. Zhåang, Yéuhâuan, 1973- III.
Helme, Michael. IV. Title. V. Series.
   R601 .W568 2003
   610'.3--dc22
                                          2003018925

Published by Paradigm Publications
www.paradigm-pubs.com
Distributed by Redwing Book Company, Taos, New Mexico USA
www.redwingbooks.com

Cover design by Herb Rich III
www.richgraphicdesign.com

Council of Oriental Medical Publishers (C.O.M.P.) Designation:
Compiled from primary Chinese sources. English terminology from Wiseman N.,
A Practical Dictionary of Chinese Medicine, Paradigm Publications, Taos, New Mexico

All rights reserved. No part of this publication may be reproduced, stored in a retrieval system or transmitted in any form by any means, electronic, mechanical, photocopying, recording or otherwise, without the prior written permission of the publisher.

Table of Contents

Preface	v
Introduction	1
Basic Vocabulary	27

1. 天 〔天〕 tiān, Heaven — 28
2. 人 〔人〕 rén, Human — 30
3. 地 〔地〕 dì, Earth — 32
4. 一 〔一〕 yī, One — 34
5. 二 〔二〕 èr, Two — 36
6. 三 〔三〕 sān, Three — 38
7. 四 〔四〕 sì, Four — 40
8. 五 〔五〕 wǔ, Five — 42
9. 六 〔六〕 liù, Six — 44
10. 七 〔七〕 qī, Seven — 46
11. 八 〔八〕 bā, Eight — 48
12. 九 〔九〕 jiǔ, Nine — 50
13. 十 〔十〕 shí, Ten — 52
14. 大 〔大〕 dà, Large — 54
15. 小 〔小〕 xiǎo, Small — 56
16. 中 〔中〕 zhōng, Center — 58
17. 上 〔上〕 shàng, Up — 60
18. 下 〔下〕 xià, Down — 62
19. 内 〔内〕 nèi, Internal — 64
20. 外 〔外〕 wài, External — 66
21. 表 〔表〕 biǎo, Exterior — 68
22. 里 〔裡〕 lǐ, Interior — 70
23. 清 〔清〕 qīng, Clear — 72
24. 浊 〔濁〕 zhuó, Turbid — 74
25. 虚 〔虛〕 xū, Vacuity — 76
26. 实 〔實〕 shí, Repletion — 78
27. 阴 〔陰〕 yīn, Yīn — 80
28. 阳 〔陽〕 yáng, Yáng — 82
29. 行 〔行〕 xíng, Phase — 84
30. 木 〔木〕 mù, Wood — 86
31. 火 〔火〕 huǒ, Fire — 88
32. 土 〔土〕 tǔ, Earth (soil) — 90
33. 金 〔金〕 jīn, Metal — 92
34. 水 〔水〕 shuǐ, Water — 94
35. 生 〔生〕 shēng, Engender — 96
36. 克 〔剋〕 kè, Restrain — 98
37. 气 〔氣〕 qì, Qì — 100
38. 血 〔血〕 xuè, Blood — 102
39. 津 〔津〕 jīn, Liquid — 104
40. 液 〔液〕 yè, Humor — 106
41. 精 〔精〕 jīng, Essence — 108
42. 神 〔神〕 shén, Spirit — 110
43. 脏 〔臟〕 zàng, Viscera — 112
44. 腑 〔腑〕 fǔ, Bowels — 114
45. 肝 〔肝〕 gān, Liver — 116
46. 心 〔心〕 xīn, Heart — 118
47. 脾 〔脾〕 pí, Spleen — 120
48. 肺 〔肺〕 fèi, Lung — 122
49. 肾 〔腎〕 shèn, Kidney — 124
50. 肠 〔腸〕 cháng, Intestine — 126
51. 胆 〔膽〕 dǎn, Gallbladder — 128
52. 胃 〔胃〕 wèi, Stomach — 130
53. 膀 〔膀〕 páng, Bladder — 132
54. 胱 〔胱〕 guāng, Bladder — 134
55. 焦 〔焦〕 jiāo, Burn(er) — 136
56. 包 〔包〕 bāo, Envelop — 138
57. 主 〔主〕 zhǔ, Govern — 140
58. 筋 〔筋〕 jīn, Sinew — 142
59. 脉 〔脈〕 mài, Vessel — 144
60. 肉 〔肉〕 ròu, Flesh — 146
61. 肌 〔肌〕 jī, Flesh — 148
62. 皮 〔皮〕 pí, Skin — 150
63. 毛 〔毛〕 máo, Body Hair — 152
64. 骨 〔骨〕 gǔ, Bone — 154
65. 窍 〔竅〕 qiào, Orifice — 156
66. 开 〔開〕 kāi, Open — 158
67. 于 〔于〕 yú, At — 160

68. 目 〔目〕	*mù*, Eye	162
69. 舌 〔舌〕	*shé*, Tongue	164
70. 口 〔口〕	*kǒu*, Mouth	166
71. 鼻 〔鼻〕	*bí*, Nose	168
72. 耳 〔耳〕	*ěr*, Ear	170
73. 经 〔經〕	*jīng*, Channel	172
74. 络 〔絡〕	*luò*, Network	174
75. 面 〔面〕	*miàn*, Face	176
76. 色 〔色〕	*sè*, Color	178
77. 青 〔青〕	*qīng*, Green-Blue	180
78. 赤 〔赤〕	*chì*, Red	182
79. 黄 〔黃〕	*huáng*, Yellow	184
80. 白 〔白〕	*bái*, White	186
81. 黑 〔黑〕	*hēi*, Black	188
82. 泪 〔淚〕	*lèi*, Tears	190
83. 汗 〔汗〕	*hàn*, Sweat	192
84. 涎 〔涎〕	*xián*, Drool	194
85. 涕 〔涕〕	*tì*, Snivel	196
86. 唾 〔唾〕	*tuò*, Spittle	198
87. 因 〔因〕	*yīn*, Cause	200
88. 邪 〔邪〕	*xié*, Evil	202
89. 淫 〔淫〕	*yín*, Excess	204
90. 风 〔風〕	*fēng*, Wind	206
91. 寒 〔寒〕	*hán*, Cold	208
92. 暑 〔暑〕	*shǔ*, Summerheat	210
93. 湿 〔濕〕	*shī*, Dampness	212
94. 燥 〔燥〕	*zào*, Dryness	214
95. 热 〔熱〕	*rè*, Heat	216
96. 温 〔溫〕	*wēn*, Warm	218
97. 痰 〔痰〕	*tán*, Phlegm	220
98. 饮 〔飲〕	*yǐn*, Drink, Rheum	222
99. 食 〔食〕	*shí*, Eat, Food	224
100. 瘀 〔瘀〕	*yū*, Stasis	226
Bibliography		229
Pinyin Index		231
English Index		232
Character Stroke Index		233

Preface

Over recent years we have witnessed a considerable growth in the number of students and practitioners of Chinese medicine who are learning Chinese. Clearly this new trend is due to growing recognition that a command of the Chinese language provides the only means of access to greater and more accurate knowledge of East Asian medicine. As the number of students of Chinese medicine continues to grow so too does the percentage of those students who demand more such access than is afforded by the current body of English literature on the subject.

This trend is reflected in a nascent body of material intended to help students who are learning Chinese with the specific goal of gaining access to Chinese medical texts. Students already have *Learn to Read Chinese* by Paul Unschuld. and *Teach Yourself to Read Modern Medical Chinese* by Bob Flaws. More recently, we have added our *Chinese Medical Chinese: Grammar and Vocabulary*. These books all focus on the vocabulary and expressions of Chinese medicine.

Nevertheless, no language-learning material so far published has emphasized introducing students to the commonly used characters of Chinese medicine in detail. This book aims to fill that gap.

Chinese is not as difficult a language as is often thought. The grammar has its complexities but is far easier than that of many Western languages. The pronunciation poses the difficulty of tonality, which is virtually absent from Western European languages. But the more daunting problem lies in mastering the script, and the materials created for learning Chinese medical Chinese so far have tended to leave the problems of character composition aside. It is true that students can find literature on this subject in the corpus of general Chinese learning aids. Nevertheless, students learning Chinese medical Chinese would benefit considerably, particularly in the initial stages of learning, if material were available that catered specifically to their needs.

The present book forms part of a series that we are creating to meet the needs of Chinese medical students. In addition to this volume on the basic vocabulary of Chinese medicine, Volume 2 will cover characters used in acupuncture point names, Volume 3 will cover the names of medicinals, Volume 4 will cover the four examinations, and Volume 5 will cover methods of treatment. Each book will introduce approximately 100 new characters, and each of Volumes 2 through 5 will presuppose a knowledge of only the characters in this volume. Once students have mastered the 100 characters in this book, they can decide which of the other character books is of most interest to them. Once all or most of these 500 characters are mastered, one can proceed to *Chinese Medical Chinese: Grammar and Vocabulary*, published by Paradigm Publications in 2002.

The Chinese script is not easy to learn, and the matter is complicated by the fact that one now has to learn two forms of it. In the People's Republic of China, the composition of many characters has been simplified to facilitate learning and enable people to write faster. The traditional complex characters continue to be used in Táiwān and Hong Kong. Although the People's Republic of China dominates the cultural life of the Chinese-speaking world and leads in the field of Chinese medicine, many Westerners start by learning the complex characters rather than the simplified characters. There are two reasons for this. One is that the historical dimension of Chinese medicine and the study of ancient texts makes Chinese medicine an area in which, even in the PRC, complex characters cannot entirely be dispensed with, so anyone wishing to study Chinese medicine in any depth through the medium of Chinese eventually needs to have a command of the complex script. The other reason is that it is generally believed Westerners can learn the simplified script more easily after having learned the complex, for reasons that will become clearer as one grasps the character explanations in this book.

In view of these considerations, we have decided that in this volume we would include both simplified and complex characters, and leave students to decide whether to learn one, the other, or both.

Thanks go to Féng Yè for reviewing the manuscript.

Introduction

Why Learn Chinese?

Learning Chinese is very probably the most rewarding single investment that a student of East Asian medicine can make. A knowledge of Chinese provides access to the knowledge and experience of East Asian physicians over a period of two thousand years. By learning Chinese, one gains entry into a library of information a thousand times larger than any that exists in English or any other Western language. One gains the ability to communicate with Chinese physicians in their own language and to share their knowledge and experience. Ultimately, one gains the ability to think in the language that has been used by generations of Chinese doctors and scholars to record their experiences and considerations about traditional Chinese medicine.

The study of primary East Asian literature has untold benefits for clinical proficiency, and learning Chinese facilitates this study. Understandably, these benefits are still often underestimated. As East Asian medicine establishes itself as a recognized profession, there is a tendency to believe that the education schools provide is complete, and therefore equal to the education provided by schools in China, Korea, or Japan. The fact is that the basis for education largely lies in literature, and there is far less literature available in the English language than in Chinese, Korean, or Japanese. Some English literature has been translated and compiled from primary East Asian sources, but much of it is based on secondary English sources and Western experience and does not fully represent the East Asian traditions. As East Asian medicine has gained root in the West, it has undergone various adaptations that have the stamp of neither scientific approval nor Asian authenticity. Learning Chinese offers students access to primary sources and enables them to get information most directly from the source, without fear of anything having been lost in the translation and transmission processes.

Students, teachers, and practitioners have another practical reason for learning Chinese. With the continual rise in standards of education that comes as the professional practice of East Asian medicine gains root in Western countries, there are already signs that Chinese-language study in the future will take on increasing importance in advanced and even regular studies and that a knowledge of Chinese will become an increasingly required qualification for teaching positions. Schools of East Asian medicine in English-speaking countries are already starting to realize the benefits of learning Chinese, so the study of Chinese language has a growing role in curricula. As this trend gains momentum, linguistic access to literature in East Asian languages, in particular Chinese, will increasingly be considered not just a luxury but a requirement for advanced studies and teaching posts, a guarantee of orthodox practice, and a hallmark of achievement.

Whether your interest is in Chinese medicine or the medical traditions of Korea or Japan, learning Chinese is essential. The Korean and Japanese traditions are built on the Chinese, and their medical terminology is essentially Chinese.

The investment required to learn Chinese may have been exaggerated in the past. Unlike other European languages such as French or Italian, Chinese has its own script, which is known to be highly complex. It is less widely known that the grammar of Chinese is infinitely much simpler than most European languages, and it has a basic structure similar to that of English. Though the script is difficult to learn, the number of characters that one has to learn for the purposes of gaining access to East Asian medical literature is astoundingly low. To master basic Chinese medical terminology one must know about 1,500 characters, the vast majority of which commonly appear in modern non-medial literature (e.g., newspapers). Nevertheless, beginning students are encouraged to find that by learning the most commonly used few hundred characters first, they can soon understand large tracts of text. Although to read Chinese medical texts with fluency one must probably know about 3,000 characters, most of these have a much lower frequency of appearance. Learning Chinese characters is difficult at first, but once one has mastered a few hundred, one acquires the ability to memorize new characters much more quickly. Thus, the purpose of the present volume and the other volumes in the Chinese Medical Characters Series is to help students over the initial hurdle.

The Nature of Chinese Language

What we call Chinese is more correctly characterized as a large group of dialects than as a single language. At the present time, Mandarin is the native dialect of the entire northern part of China as well as of the southwest. The subdialect specific to Běijīng is the lingua franca of the Chinese world and hence is the dialect most commonly learned by non-Chinese. South of a line that roughly corresponds with the Chángjiāng (Yangtze River) and east of Sìchuān and Guìzhōu are the dialects of the southeast, including the Wú dialect of Shànghǎi and the Zhèjiāng region, the Gàn dialects of Jiāngxī, the Xiāng dialects of Húnán, the Mǐn dialects of Fújiàn and Táiwān, the Yuè dialects of Guǎngdōng and Guǎngxī, and the Kèjiā (Hakka) dialects of the region of the border between Fújiàn and Guǎngdōng.

These dialects together form the Chinese branch of the Sino-Tibetan family of languages. Many other languages not belonging to the Sino-Tibetan family are spoken among the minority groups largely located in northwestern and southwestern China. These include Korean, Mongolian, Turkic, Tibeto-Burman, Tai, Miao-Yao, Bai, Mon-Khmer, and Austronesian languages. They have influenced and have been influenced by Chinese, but they do not concern us here.

The dialects of Chinese are not all mutually intelligible. They have been traditionally called 方言 *fāng yán* (literally "place" + "speech") in China because of their close relationship, and this term has been equated with our English word "dialect." But when a native of Běijīng travels to Shànghǎi, Chángshā, Nánchāng, Guǎngzhōu, or Xiàmén, he does not understand the local dialects at all. In reality, they are distinct but very similar languages, comparable in terms of both similarity and difference to many European languages such as Danish, Norwegian, and Swedish.

Many of the words in each dialect are cognates, though they often differ so widely in pronunciation as to be almost unrecognizable in an unfamiliar dialect. The first person pronoun is *wǒ* in Mandarin, *ngou* in Wú, *guà* in Mǐn, and *ngǒ* in Yuè. Our European languages also have many cognates. The word for *I* is *je* in French, *io* in Italian, *yo* in Spanish, *ego* in Latin, *ich* in German, and *jeg* in Danish. All these are cognate words, although in fact we might never recognize them before actually learning the languages in question. In the Chinese dialects, a large proportion of the words used are cognates. There are many unique words in each, but most are similar.

There are great similarities in the grammar of all the dialects. For example, they all have a basic subject-verb-object word-order in simple sentences, just as our own language has. In this pattern, qualifiers generally precede what they qualify, i.e., adjectives precede nouns, and adverbs precede verbs.

An essential feature of the Chinese dialects is that in fact words do not change their form according to grammatical function in the way words in English and other European languages do. As we shall see, this has considerable consequences. Our languages change the form of nouns to mark the plural (cat/cats, foot/feet); they change the form of verbs to mark person and tense (show/shows/showed/shown). These changes are called inflexions, and hence European languages are described as being inflexional in nature. The Chinese dialects, by contrast, do not share this feature. They express all the features expressed in English by modifying words—as far as there are parallels—with separate words. Chinese nouns are not marked for plurality, and whether a word is singular or plural is indicated by a numeral or otherwise left to be inferred from context. Chinese verbs indicate only actions; the time of the action is indicated, if at all, by other words in the sentence. Chinese considers the basic meaning of words to be separate, or isolated, from concepts such as plurality and tense. It is therefore characterized as an isolating language.

A further feature of Chinese, which is observed in the historical dimension, is the gradual development from monosyllablism to polysyllablism. Even today, the smallest unit of sound and meaning in Chinese is the single syllable. As in the past, each syllable is represented by a single character (or graph, as it is sometimes known). In ancient Chinese texts, each character roughly corresponds to a word in English. There are many compound nouns, but for the most part, the elements of compounds can stand as independent words. A language in which distinct words are monosyllabic must have a wide range of monosyllabic sounds if words are to be distinguished. This was the case of Old Chinese, the language spoken up till the Hàn dynasty (the early part of the first millennium in our own chronological terms). Toward the end of the Old Chinese period, Chinese was undergoing a considerable reduction in the number of its overall sounds, which meant that a single syllable was no longer sufficient to distinguish words. For example, ear in ancient Chinese was expressed as *ěr,* but in the modern spoken Mandarin, it is expressed in a compound as *ěr duo* "ear flower." Because the literature and terminology of Chinese medicine spans two thousand years of development, we see considerable variation in expression due to greater or lesser tendencies toward compounding at different stages in the language.

A final feature of Chinese to be mentioned is its script. Before providing a detailed description of the writing system, we should examine its essential nature in relation to the language as a whole.

English and other European languages familiar to readers are essentially phonetic. The letters of the alphabet are used to represent sounds. English is a poor example of phonetic writing, because many of our spellings have not been updated to represent the sounds of the modern language. Spanish and German are markedly more phonetic, in the sense that once one knows what sounds are ascribed to individual letters of the alphabet and combinations of them, one can pronounce almost any word. English, by contrast, does not have anything like a one-to-one correspondence between sound and written sign. For example, 'buy,' 'by,' and 'bi-' are homophones written differently. 'Read' on the other hand represents two distinct sounds depending on whether the present or the past tense is intended.

Chinese differs from European languages in that it has graphs that represent words, rather than the sounds composing them. The Chinese script is therefore call logographic (logos is simply the Greek for word). Although many Chinese characters contain a phonetic element, the script is not fundamentally phonetic.

All known scripts were originally derived from picture writing. The earliest graphic representations created by humans were direct representations of things and ideas. We speak of "writing" when graphic representations came to be used to represent spoken words in the normal sequence of language. Pictures of objects became simplified, stylized, and to a certain degree standardized. In other words, they became pictographs. However, the need to represent the non-visual aspects of human language turned the attention increasingly toward the representation of the sounds of the language.

The scripts of the Middle East, from which our Roman alphabet derives, gradually evolved so that all pictographic elements gave way to essentially phonetic representation. Chinese differs in that, although phonetic elements were incorporated, pictographic elements were never discarded.

One reason why a fully phonetic script did not develop for Chinese lies in the nature of the isolating language. The script never had to take account of inflexions, which are found in so many other languages. Differences such as between 'speak,' 'speaks,' 'spoke,' and 'spoken' are most easily catered to by a writing system that is phonetic. The absence of such differences in Chinese allowed non-phonetic characters to perform their task quite adequately.

The Chinese writing system is a complex mixture of pictographic and phonetic elements. Because each character has to be memorized, it is much more difficult to learn than a phonetic script. Nevertheless, by not being tied to sound, it has the one great advantage that it does not have to represent sound variations. Chinese characters are rather like Arabic numerals, which are now used universally even though they are read differently by speakers of different languages. The character 3, for example, is read variously as *trois* in French, *tres* in Spanish, *drei* in German, and *sān* in Chinese. In Chinese, the character 三 represents the same concept for speakers of all Chinese dialects, never mind what sound they associate with it.

This feature of the Chinese script serves as a bridge that not only spans contemporary dialects, but also different stages in the development of the language. Despite the great changes in the language, the Chinese script provides access to the literature of the past in a way that no other language does. In English, we can barely read the 14th century Middle English of Chaucer without a translation, let alone the 8th century Old English of *Beowulf*; yet a knowledge of written Chinese gives us access to the literature of two thousand years ago or earlier. Ancient texts present problems because they may contain words that have become obsolete or that, though familiar to modern speakers, no longer have the same meaning. But the existence of large amounts of words that have merely changed in pronunciation makes the reading of ancient texts possible.

The great stability of the written language means that the modern student of Chinese medicine has relatively easy access to the literature of the past. And of course the English-speaking student embarking on the task of learning Chinese can similarly gain access to the literature of the past as well as the present. The continuing importance of the classical literature of antiquity requires students to be conversant with classical as well as modern Chinese. The continuity of the written language means merely having to learn different forms of the same language rather than distinct languages.

But before proceeding with a more detailed description of the Chinese script, let us first of all introduce the pronunciation of Chinese words.

Transcription and Pronunciation

Transcription

There are a number of different ways to transcribe Chinese sounds. The one now most commonly used internationally is Hànyǔ Pīnyīn, which English speakers normally refer to as simply Pīnyīn. This was adopted by the government of the People's Republic of China in the 1950s and by the world press in the 1970s. Pīnyīn is used to teach the sounds of Mandarin in school and to indicate pronunciation in dictionaries. It was once hoped that it could replace the complex Chinese script as a part of Communist government policy to reduce bourgeois hegemony of literacy. This hope has never materialized because of the huge implications it would have for the continuity and development of the written Chinese language. However, Hànyǔ Pīnyīn is the only method used for indicating the pronunciation of characters in the PRC, and it is used to enable elementary school children to relate the sounds of speech to written characters.

Prior to the advent of Hànyǔ Pīnyīn, the most commonly used variety of transcription in the English language was the Wade-Giles system. This continued to be used by Western sinologists until the advent of the computer, when library catalogs could be updated to include both transcription systems. Wade-Giles has been retained in Táiwān, where Pīnyīn has never been adopted for political reasons (anything Communist is rejected), although there are currently moves to change this. Táiwān uses alphabetical transcription for international purposes, but it has a set of thirty seven phonetic symbols derived from Chinese characters that are used to indicate the sounds of characters (ㄅ ㄆ ㄇ ㄈ…). The Mandarin Phonetic Symbols are also used to help elementary school children relate the sounds of spoken language to written characters. A fourth Romanization system is Guoyeu Romatzyh devised by Yale University. This has never been widely used.

We might point out that before the advent of Roman transcription systems, the Chinese for centuries indicated the pronunciation of words by the *fǎn qiē* 反切 method. According to this method, the sound of a character is indicated by splicing the initial and final sounds of two other characters. Thus, the pronunciation of 水 *shuǐ* is indicated as "數軌切", or the *sh* of 數 *sh(ù)* spliced with the *uǐ* of 軌 *(g)uǐ*. This method is still used and found in certain larger dictionaries alongside modern transcriptions. It is not suitable for beginners of Chinese to use because it presumes knowledge of a large number of characters.

Pīnyīn is the most complete and accurate description of Modern Mandarin pronunciation, and it was designed with marks to indicate tones. Wade-Giles Romanization in its original form includes some distinctions that are no longer current in Modern Mandarin and traditionally included no indication of tonality, no doubt because Western scholars were traditionally uninterested in the spoken language.

All systems of transcription inherently have the disadvantage that the sound value of many letters and combinations of letters have to be learned. Without instruction, English speakers cannot produce the correct sounds. Pīnyīn has been criticized because, though geared to greater economy, certain letters represent sounds very distant from any sounds they ever represent in English (the *c* of *cai*, for example, is pronounced as *ts*).

Sounds

Accurate pronunciation in any language can only be learned from native speakers of that language. When learning Chinese, you should seek out a good native speaker of Mandarin. Standard Mandarin is spoken in Běijīng, and someone from Běijīng will provide you with the best model for pronunciation. If no courses in Mandarin are being offered in your locality or if you cannot find a good Mandarin speaker to help you with your pronunciation, you can purchase teach-yourself Chinese textbooks with tapes or CDs that teach the pronunciation. These are usually available in the larger bookstores and can be easily ordered anywhere.

Most of the sounds of Mandarin are quite easy for English speakers to reproduce. Only a few are difficult. Never be afraid to ask Chinese people to help you learn how to pronounce words. They generally give encouragement to anyone learning their language and always tell you how good your pronunciation is!

In what follows, the sounds of Mandarin are explained in rough English equivalents. Sounds in other European languages are given where they are closer to the Chinese sounds. In some cases, phonetic symbols have been added in brackets, e.g., [æ], [ɑ], to clarify the value of certain sounds.

b   Like the English *b,* but unaspirated, so that it actually sounds more like the *p* in *spay.* The Chinese 八 *bā,* meaning 'eight', resembles the *ba* in "Ba, ba, black sheep"; 痹 *bì,* 'impediment', sounds like the English *bee*.

p   Like the English *p*, but well aspirated such as when uttering the word *pig* as an invective (as in "You pig!"). The Chinese 脾 *pí,* 'spleen', resembles the *p* in *pea*. Note that in English *b* and *p* are distinguished in normal speech by the presence and absence of voicing, while in Chinese they are distinguished by the absence and presence of aspiration. A similar difference exists between *d* and *t* and between *g* and *k*.[1]

---

[1] Wade-Giles transcription represented the unaspirated sounds as p, t, k and the aspirated sounds as p', t', k'. This difference in transcription system explains why Dao and Daoism used to be written as Tao and Taoism, and why *dāng guī* was borrowed into English in the form tangkuei.

m	As the English *m*. The Chinese 母 *mǔ*, 'mother', is pronounced like *moo*, the sound made by a cow.
f	Exactly as the English *f*. Thus 非 *fēi*, 'not', sounds like the name *Fay*.
d	Roughly as the *d* of the English *dog*, but unaspirated, so that it actually sounds more like the *t* in *stow*. The Chinese 斗 *dǒu*, 'to shake', is pronounced like the English *doe* (a female deer).
t	Roughly as the *t* of the English *ten*, but more strongly aspirated. (It is never pronounced as the *t* in the American English *better*.) Thus the Chinese 头 *tóu*, 'head', resembles the *t* in *tow*; 土 *tǔ*, 'earth' or 'soil', resembles the English *two*; 体 *tǐ*, 'body', resembles the English *tea*.
l	Initial l-, as in 累 *lèi*, 'tired', which sounds like the English *lay*.
n	As the English *n*. The Chinese 内 *nèi*, 'inside', is pronounced like the archaic English *nay*; 脑 *nǎo*, 'brain', sounds like the English *now*; 逆 *nì*, 'counterflow', sounds like the English *knee*.
g	As the English *g* in *get* (not as the *g* of *genial*). Thus, the Chinese 根 *gēn*, 'root', resembles the English *gun*. The Chinese *g* sound is unaspirated and sounds more like the *k* in *skin*.
k	As the English *k*, though more strongly aspirated. The Chinese 哭 *kū*, 'to weep', sounds similar to the English *coo*; 开 *kāi* sounds like the *ki* of *kite*.
h	Approximately as the English *h*, so that 黑 *hēi*, 'black', resembles *hay*. A characteristic of good Mandarin, however, is a tendency toward a slight rasping sound like the *ch* in the Scottish pronunciation of *loch* or the German *Bach*, or like the *j* in the Spanish *jamón*.
j	Approximately as the *j* in *judge* or the *g* in *gemini*. Thus 悸 *jì*, 'palpitations', is pronounced like *gee*. If one listens carefully to native Mandarin speakers, one finds that the sound is not voiced like the English sound. The *j* in Pīnyīn is always followed by an *i* or by a *u* pronounced as [ü]. Examples include: 降 *jiàng*, 'downbear', 结 *jié*, 'bind', 紧 *jǐn*, 'tight', 灸 *jiǔ*, 'moxibustion', 疽 *jū*, 'flat-abscess', 卷 *juǎn*, 'curled', and 君 *jūn*, 'sovereign'.
q	As the *ch* in cheese. The Chinese 气 *qì*, meaning 'qì' or 'air', is pronounced like the *chee* in *cheek*. Like *j*, *q* is followed by *i* or by *u* pronounced as [ü]. Examples include: 掐 *qiā*, 'fingernail pressing', 欠 *qiàn*, 'lack', 秋 *qiū*, 'autumn', 清 *qīng*, 'clear', 曲 *qū*, 'fermented leaven', 去 *qù*, 'remove', and 全 *quán*, 'complete'.

x	Similar to the English *sh*, so that 细 *xì*, 'thin' or 'fine', resembles the English *she*. However, if you listen to Chinese speakers, you will discover that the sound is wispier than the English *sh*, so that *xì* sounds nearly as much like the English *see* as the English *she*. The *x* in Pīnyīn is always followed by an *i* or a *u* pronounced as [ü]. Examples: 下 *xià*, 'down', 泄 *xiè*, 'discharge', 涎 *xián*, 'drool', 胸 *xiōng*, 'chest', 羞 *xiū*, 'be shy of', 'aversion to', 心 *xīn*, 'heart', 虚 *xū*, 'vacuity', 循 *xún*, 'feel (one's way)', and 宣 *xuān*, 'diffuse'.
zh	As the *j* in the English *jowl*, but curling the tongue backward to make an *r* sound. Unlike the English *j* sound, the Chinese *zh* is not voiced. One example is 针 *zhēn*, 'needle', pronounced something like the last syllable of the English *dungeon*.
ch	As the *ch* in *cheese,* but curling the tongue backward to make an *r* sound. Unlike the English *ch* sound, the Chinese *ch* is not voiced. This sound occurs in 尺 *chǐ*, 'cubit', 肠 *cháng*, 'intestine', 潮 *cháo*, 'tidal', 冲 *chōng,* 'thoroughfare', and 喘 *chuǎn*, 'panting'.
sh	Produced like the *sh* in *ship*, but curling the tongue backward to make an *r* sound. This sound occurs in 疝 *shàn*, 'mounting', 伤 *shāng*, 'damage', 少 *shào*, 'lesser', 肾 *shèn*, 'kidney', 湿 *shī*, 'dampness', 手 *shǒu*, 'hand', and 水 *shuǐ*, 'water'.
r	As the *r* in *road*, but in some circumstances tending toward the sound of *g* in *beige*. The Chinese 肉 *ròu*, 'flesh', sounds like the English *roe*; 乳 *rǔ*, 'breast', sounds like the English *rue*. Other examples include 软 *ruǎn*, 'soft', 弱 *ruò*, 'weak', and 人 *rén*, 'human'.
z	As the *ds* in *heads*. The Chinese 杂 *zá*, 'miscellaneous', sounds like the *za* in *mozzarella* when pronounced by an Italian. This sound also occurs in 足 *zú*, 'foot', and 滋 *zī*, 'enrich'.
c	As the *ts* in *Whitsun*. This is also like the German *z,* as in *Zeitgeist*. This sound occurs in 刺 *cì,* 'to needle'.
s	As the *s* in *see*, never as the *s* in *easy*. Occurs in 三 *sān*, 'three', 四 *sì*, 'four', and 色 *sè*, 'color'.
-i, y	The final *-i* is pronounced in two different ways. 1) After *z-, c-,* and *s-* and after the retroflex sounds *zh-, ch-, sh-,* and *r-*, it is barely pronounced at all. For instance, *zi* is pronounced as '*dzzz*' with virtually no vowel except for a brief continuation of the voice as the teeth part after producing the '*z*' sound.

Examples include 子 *zǐ*, 'child', 'son', 刺 *cì*, 'to needle', and 思 *sī*, 'thought'. Examples of the post-retroflex *i* include 肢 *zhī*, 'limb', 迟 *chí*, 'slow', 食 *shí*, 'food', and 日 *rì*, 'sun'. 2) After other consonants, it sounds like the *ee* in the English *see*. Thus, 淋 *lín*, 'strangury', sounds like the English *lean*, though shorter. Other examples include 病 *bìng*, 'disease', 津 *jīn*, 'liquid', 情 *qíng*, 'affect'. The sound *yi*, which occurs in the initial position only, is pronounced as the archaic English pronoun *ye*. Before *ao, an, ang, u,* and *e*, it is pronounced as the English *y*, e.g., 表 *biǎo*, 'exterior', 跷 *qiāo*, 'springing (vessel)', 钱 *qián*, 'money', 'qián (weight)', 点 *diǎn*, 'speckle', 绛 *jiàng*, 'crimson', 久 *jiǔ*, 'for a long time' or 'enduring', 跌 *dié*, 'fall', and 液 *yè*, 'humor'.

-u, w The final *u* is pronounced as the *oo* in *food* or as the *o* in *do*. More precisely it is like the *u* in the German *nu* or Spanish *su*, since the rounding of the lips is kept the same throughout the syllable. Examples include 母 *mǔ*, 'mother', 毒 *dú*, 'poison', 补 *bǔ*, 'supplement', 浮 *fú*, 'floating', 腑 *fǔ*, 'bowel', 腹 *fù*, 'abdomen', 颅 *lù*, 'skull', 骨 *gǔ*, 'bone', 谷 *gǔ*, 'grain', 固 *gù*, 'secure', 主 *zhǔ*, 'govern', 搐 *chù*, 'convulsions', 暑 *shǔ*, 'summerheat', and 促 *cù*, 'skipping'. When -*u* is not the last sound in the syllable, it is pronounced as the English *w*, e.g., 酸 *suān*, 'sour', 窜 *cuàn*, 'scurry', 乱 *luàn*, 'chaotic', 短 *duǎn*, 'short', 光 *guāng*, 'light', 滑 *huá*, 'slippery', 化 *huà*, 'transform', and 黄 *huáng*, 'yellow'. When this sound occurs as an initial, it is written as *w*, e.g., 五 *wǔ*, 'five', 脘 *wǎn*, 'stomach duct'. Finally, the combination *ui* is pronounced as the English *way* (not as the English *we*).[2] Examples include 回 *huí*, 'return', 归 *guī*, 'return', 水 *shuǐ*, 'water', and 睡 *shuì*, 'sleep'.

-ü, -u, yu The final –*ü*, as 去 *qù*, 'to go', or 绿 *lǜ*, 'green', pronounced like a French *u* or a German *ü*, that is often represented as [ü] in phonetic scripts. No equivalent of this sound exists in English except in the Scottish pronunciation of the vowel sound appearing in choose or lute. This sound is spelled as *ü* (with an umlaut on the *u*) after *l* or *n*, e.g., 女 *nǚ*, 'female', or 绿 *lǜ*, 'green', to distinguish the sound from the *u* representing the English *oo* [u]. The umlaut is not used when the sound of the initial is *j, q, x,* or *y*; in this position it is always pronounced as [ü], never as [u].

---

[2] The convention of using *ui* to represent a sound similar to the English *way* is apparently explicable in terms of economy of letters. Older transcriptions represented the sound, somewhat more clearly, as *uei*, as in the English loanword tangkuei.

Examples include: 菊 *jú*, 'chrysanthemum', 曲 *qū*, 'fermented leaven', 倦 *juàn*, 'fatigued', 蜷 *quán*, 'curled-up', 血 *xuè*, 'blood', 元 *yuán*, 'origin', 晕 *yūn*, 'dizziness', and 运 *yùn*, 'move'.

a As the *a* in French, Spanish, or Italian (or in the Northern English pronunciation of *grass*). It is often represented in phonetic notation as [ɑ]. It is like the *a* in *father*, but shorter and more open. It is not pronounced like the *a* in *bad*. Examples include 八 *bā*, 'eight', 发 *fā*, 'effuse', 法 *fǎ*, 'method', and 大 *dà*, 'great'.

-o, -uo, wo The final *-o* sounds like *awe* in the British rather than the American pronunciation. This sound can directly follow *b, p, m,* and *f,* e.g., 剥 *bō*, 'peeling' (tongue fur), 薄 *bó*, 'thin', 破 *pò*, 'break', 磨 *mó*, 'grind', and 佛 *fó*, 'Buddha'. After all other initials (*d, t, n, l, h, zh, ch, sh, r, z, c,* and *s*) *o* does not occur alone, but it is preceded by *u* and sounds like the *wa* of *war* in the British pronunciation. Examples include 多 *duō*, 'much', 脱 *tuō*, 'shed', 'desertion', 络 *luò*, 'network vessel', 火 *huǒ*, 'fire', 浊 *zhuó*, 'turbid', 说 *shuō*, 'dictum', 弱 *ruò*, 'weak', 左 *zuǒ*, 'left', 错 *cuò*, 'cross', and 所 *suǒ*, 'place'. The same sound occurring in the initial position is written as *wo*, as in 我 *wǒ*, 'I', 'me'.

e The Pīnyīn *e* is used to represent two distinct sounds. Final *-e*, after *i* or *u*, like the *e* in *bed* [ɛ]. In all other positions, it is like the vowel in bird without any *r* sound, or like œ in the French *hors d'œuvre*, a sound which is often represented in phonetic notation as [œ]. Examples: 阿 *ē* of 阿胶 *ē jiāo*, 'ass-hide glue', 蛾 *é*, 'moth', 恶 *è*, 'malign', 得 *dé*, 'obtain', 膈 *gé*, 'diaphragm', 和 *hé*, 'harmonize', 克 *kè*, 'restrain'.

ai As the English *eye* (actually more closely to the German *ei* of *Heim*). It occurs in 艾 *ài*, 'moxa', 'mugwort', 脉 *mài*, 'vessel', 'pulse', 苔 *tāi*, 'tongue fur', and 开 *kāi*, 'open'.

ei As the *ei* in the English feint. The Chinese 胃 *wèi*, 'stomach', is pronounced as the English *weigh* or *way*, while 累 *lèi*, 'tired', sounds like the English *lay*. Other examples include 黑 *hēi*, 'black', 肥 *féi*, 'obese', and 肺 *fèi*, 'lung'.

ao As the *ow* of *how*. Thus, 脑 *nǎo*, 'brain', is pronounced more or less like the English *now*. In actual fact, the sound is closer to the *au* of the German *Haus* or the Spanish *jaula*. Another example is 膏 *gāo*, 'unctuous' (as in 膏淋 *gāo lín*, 'unctuous strangury').

ou As the English *oh!*, especially in the American pronunciation rather than the standard British pronunciation. This sound can occur in the initial position, as in 呕 *ǒu*, 'retching', which sounds like *oh!* It more often occurs as a final, as in 抽 *chōu*, 'tug', 稠 *chóu*, 'thick', 'viscous', 腠 *còu*, 'interstice', 漏 *lòu*, 'to leak', 'spotting', 痘 *dòu*, 'pox', 喉 *hóu*, 'larynx', 厚 *hòu*, 'thick', 后 *hòu*, 'after', and 垢 *gòu*, 'grimy'.

an As the *an* in the Spanish word *pan* meaning *bread*. The *n* sound tends to be rather nasal and indistinct. It occurs in 安 *ān*, 'to quiet', 寒 *hán*, 'cold', 烦 *fán*, 'vexation', 反 *fǎn*, 're(flux)' (as in 反胃 *fǎn wèi*, 'stomach reflux'), 肝 *gān*, 'liver', 甘 *gān*, 'sweet', 满 *mǎn*, 'fullness', and 缓 *huǎn*, 'moderate'. After *xi, xu, y,* or *i*, it is pronounced, depending on the speaker, either like the English pronunciation of *Anne* (with [æ] as the vowel sound) or as *en* in the English *yen*. Examples include 前 *qián*, 'before', 先 *xiān*, 'advanced', 'earlier', 弦 *xián*, 'stringlike', 宣 *xuán*, 'diffuse', and 蜷 *quán*, 'curled-up'.

en As the *un* of the English *undo*, with the mouth less widely opened. Thus 本 *běn*, 'root', resembles the English *bun* (never as the English name *Ben*). Similarly, 分 *fēn*, 'fēn' (a weight), is pronounced like the English *fun*. The *n* sound tends to be rather nasal and indistinct. This sound also occurs in 奔 *bēn*, 'running' (as in running piglet), and 身 *shēn*, 'body'.

ang As the *ang* in *sang*, but with the *a* pronounced like the *a* in *father* (though not so long). This sound occurs in 脏 *zàng*, 'viscus', 胀 *zhàng*, 'distention', 胖 *pàng*, 'obese', 养 *yǎng*, 'nourish', and 肠 *cháng*, 'intestine'.

eng The final *-eng* is similar to the *ung* in the English *sung*. (Beware, it is not pronounced like the *eng* in the English *length*). Thus, 崩 *bēng*, 'flooding' (metrorrhagia), is pronounced like the English *bung*, though with the mouth less widely opened. This sound also occurs in 蒸 *zhēng*, 'steam', 风 *fēng*, 'wind', 症 *zhēng*, 'concretion', and 证 *zhèng*, 'pattern'.

er The final *-er* is pronounced as the *er* in the American English *her*. Examples include 儿 *ér*, 'child', and 耳 *ěr*, 'ear'.

-r The final *-r* is a characteristic of Běijīng speech that in most cases is considered optional in Mandarin. In Chinese characters, it is represented by the character 儿 *ér*, which is a noun suffix. In speech, however, it is not pronounced as a distinct syllable, but as a rhotacization of the syllable it follows. Examples include 小孩儿 *xiǎo háir*, 'child', 开方儿 *kāi fāng ér*, 'write a prescription'. Noun forms with this ending are regularly

Chinese Medical Characters: Basic Vocabulary

heard in conversation, but seen in literature only in novels in which the author wishes to highlight speech idiosyncrasies. In Chinese medical literature, such forms are rarely seen, and other forms are used instead (e.g., 小儿 xiǎo ér, 'child'; 开处方 kāi chǔ fāng, 'write a prescription').

Tones

The notion of tonality is by no means an alien concept in English. We pronounce words with different intonation to express slight nuances in meaning such as inquiry, doubt, and affirmation. English question sentences, for example, are often characterized by a rising intonation at the end. (In "Is he coming?" the word 'coming' is usually pronounced with a rising intonation.) Chinese tones differ in that each syllable has a fixed tone that is an integral part of the pronunciation rather than an expression of nuance. Westerners usually find the tones are relatively easy to reproduce. The difficulty lies only in abandoning our native habit of varying intonation in running speech and in giving each word the correct tone.

1st Tone (第一声 dì yī shēng) A syllable in the first tone, marked as " ¯ ", has a high level sound.

2nd Tone (第二声 dì èr shēng) A syllable in the second tone, marked as " ´ ", has a high rising tone. As in the English "Yes?" or "Oh?"

3rd Tone (第三声 dì sān shēng) A syllable in the third tone, marked as " ˇ ", has a low dipping tone.

4th Tone (第四声 dì sì shēng) A syllable in the fourth tone, marked as " ` ", falls from a high level to a low level. As in the English "No!"

These tones are fixed in all cases except the third tone, which changes to a second tone when it precedes a syllable in third tone. Thus, 解表 jiě biǎo is read as jié biǎo (even though the Pīnyīn is not normally written like that).

In Modern Mandarin there is also what is called a neutral tone, which occurs in compounds that are largely confined to colloquial expression. The neutral tone, which is marked in Pīnyīn by the absence of any tone mark, is in fact not one, but two distinct tones. After a syllable in first, second, and fourth tones, a neutral tone is a low falling tone, like the first half of a full third tone, e.g., 狮子 shī zi, 'lion'; 孩子 hái zi, 'child'; 杏子 xìng zi, 'apricot'. After a third tone, it is like a first tone but slightly lower, e.g., 饺子 jiǎo zi. The noun suffix 子 zi accounts for most occurrences of the neutral tone. But the final element in certain compounds is also conventionally pronounced (especially in Běijīng) in the neutral tone. Examples include 太太 *tài tai,* 'Mrs.'; 先生 *xiān sheng,* 'Mr.'; 老鸹 *lǎo gua,* 'crow'; and 老顽固 *lǎo wán gu,* 'old stick-in-the-mud'.

Homophony

A feature of Chinese is that many of its monosyllabic words are homophonic, i.e., share the same sound. This feature stemmed from a reduction of the number of sounds in the ancient language and has resulted in two words often having to be used instead of one. (This is why, for example, 耳 *ěr* has been replaced by 耳朵 *ěr duo* in the modern spoken language.) Vast numbers of words are distinguished by tone alone, but many words have exactly the same sound and tone. The homophony of Chinese poses considerable difficulties to the foreign student learning Chinese language.

Non-Standard Pronunciation

Although China is a land of many different dialects, many of which are not mutually intelligible, Mandarin is not only taught in all elementary schools, it also provides the medium of all education throughout China and Táiwān. Whatever dialect Chinese people may learn from their parents or from their local community, most people now have a command of Mandarin that facilitates communication with anyone in the Chinese world. Nevertheless, the speech of many Chinese does not conform to standard Mandarin pronunciation and contains elements from local dialects. In particular, the retroflex sounds *zh, ch,* and *sh,* which are unique to Mandarin, are difficult for native speakers of other dialects to produce and tend to be replaced with the non-retroflex equivalents *z, c,* and *s*. This tendency is common to people as far apart as Sìchuān, Shànghǎi, Guǎngzhōu, and Táiwān. Some southern Chinese (notably Fújiànese and Táiwānese) who are not native speakers of Mandarin have difficulty making the sound *f,* and tend to pronounce it is *hw*. In addition, they often fail to distinguish *l* from *n*, pronouncing both as *n*.

Evolution of the Script

The Chinese script appears as a fully developed writing system in the late Shāng dynasty (14th to 11th centuries B.C.E.). Inscriptions on oracle bones and shells and on bronzes show a mature writing system capable of recording the contemporary Chinese language in a complete and unambiguous manner. In view of this, a long period of initial development has been suggested.

These so-called oracle-bone inscriptions were carved on the ventral shells of tortoises or on the scapulae of larger animals, such as oxen. They were the interpretation of the cracks in the shell or bone understood to answer questions about the outcomes of future events. Oracle-bone divining was a mysterious and sacred procedure performed by shamans. The shaman bored holes in the shells, then inserted a burning stick while posing the question to which an answer was sought. The heat caused cracks to appear, and these cracks were believed to be the encrypted answer to the question posed. The information obtained from the cracks in the bones and tortoise shells was written down in a way that both recorded the patterns of the cracks and arranged them into meaningful arrays that included the shaman's interpretations. It is believed that the script found on oracle shells and bones was first developed specifically for noting oracle interpretations and was later extended to other uses.

Graphs and Etymology

Chinese etymology is far from a science. Sinologists could debate for decades over the origins of certain characters and never come to a final resolution. Students learning Chinese for the purpose of understanding Chinese medicine could mistakenly think of etymology as a specialty field of little professional interest to themselves. But investing some time in the study of the roots of characters not only facilitates memorization of those characters, it also helps the student develop a deeper understanding of the patterns of thought and expression that are implicit in the language and therefore the literature of Chinese medicine.

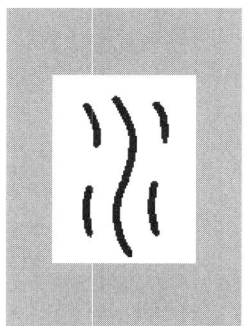

As has already been pointed out, the Chinese writing system was originally pictographic. In their original forms, graphs representing animals and objects were self-explanatory. For ease of writing, however, the pictographs were simplified and stylized, so that the referents are sometimes not easily recognized. Water is a good example; the original character looks like water (see illustration), whereas the stylized versions 水 and 氵 do not.

Not all elements of the language could be represented in pictorial form. Other devices had to be used. Some notions could be represented in an abstract fashion, as for example the graphs 上 *shàng* and 下 *xià*, meaning up and down; these characters are said to be ideographic. Pictographs could also be combined, such as the combination of 日 *rì*, sun, and 月 *yuè*, moon, which forms 明 *míng* and represents *bright* or *brightness*; characters like this are said to be "associative compounds."

What could be achieved in these ways was also limited, and ultimately the easiest way of representing many elements of the language was to evoke the sounds of the words in speech.

One way of doing this was simply to borrow a word of similar sound. Because this method led to the existence of confusing homographs, confusion was avoided by combining the phonetic loan with another element, known as a signific or radical, that roughly represented the sphere of meaning. Thus, 工 (now pronounced *gōng*) was borrowed to represent the similar-sounding word for 'river', but combined with the water signific to form 江 (now pronounced *jiāng*). In similar fashion, 干 (now pronounced *gān*), shield, was combined with the flesh signific 肉 (simplified to 月) to form 肝, which represents the liver (now pronounced *gān*); 干 was also combined with the water signific 水 (simplified to 氵) to form 汗, which is used to represent sweat (now pronounced *hàn*). This method of combining significs and phonetics came to be the most productive method of creating characters; characters thus created are called "signific-phonetic compounds."

The four types of characters mentioned in the preceding paragraphs (i.e., pictographs, ideographs, associative compounds, and signific-phonetic compounds) explain characters in terms of their formation. But Chinese etymologists speak of two other categories that are based on how the characters are used. One category, 转注 *zhuǎn zhù*, mutually interpretive, has been explained in several ways. The most common explanation is that it refers to words sharing the same signific that are synonymous with and can explain each other, such as 老 *lǎo* (meaning 'old age') and 考 *kǎo* (which originally meant 'long life' or 'aged', but which has come to mean 'to test'). The other category is called 假借 *jiǎ jiè,* loan characters, which are words that are taken from one context and used, mostly for their pronunciation, in an entirely different context. For example, 來 *lái* was originally a pictograph of 'wheat' or 'corn' and was later borrowed to represent 'come.'

Below is a table that reviews the different categories of Chinese graphs and the descriptions of character composition by which each of the characters in this book is classified. For some categories, once the image or concept represented in the characters is pointed out, they will naturally be retained in one's memory. This most often happens with the pictographs and ideographs, as well as with certain associative compounds. In other cases it may be more time efficient to remember the character by rote (or by associating their significs and/or phonetics with other characters) rather than by trying to rely on obscure mnemonic clues.

Categories of Chinese Graphs			
Category Name		**Translation**	**Examples**
Simplified	Complex		
象形	〔象形〕	*xiàng xíng*, pictographs	日 *rì*, sun; 月 *yuè*, moon; 木 *mù*, tree;	山 *shān*, mountain; 子 *zǐ*, child; 女 *nǚ*, girl, woman
指事	〔指事〕	*zhǐ shì*, ideographs/ indicators	一 *yī*, one; 二 *èr*, two	上 *shàng*, up; 下 *xià*, down
形声	〔形聲〕	*xíng shēng*, signific-phonetic compounds		江 *jiāng*, river; 汗 *hàn*, sweat
会意	〔會意〕	*huì yì*, associative compounds	子 + 女 = 好 *hào*, like, love	日 + 月 = 明 *míng*, brightness
转注	〔轉注〕	*zhuǎn zhù*, mutually interpretive	老 *lǎo*, old age	考 *kǎo*, originally long life, now test
假借	〔假借〕	*jiǎ jiè*, loan characters		来 *lái*, come

Graphs and Dictionary Usage

As explained above, Chinese characters are not all arbitrary symbols. Most of them are composed of elements that are found over and over again in different characters. One element of the character is designated as the key element, or signific, which represents the basic category of meaning. Examples of this include: most characters denoting herbs have the grass signific 艹 (which at an earlier stage was written as 艸, depicting small plants); most trees and objects made of wood have the tree/wood signific 木 among their parts; liquids and things to do with liquids mostly have the water signific 氵; most characters denoting disease names have the sickbed signific 疒. Examples of characters in which these and other significs appear are given below.

氵 ***shuǐ*, water signific:** 汗 *hàn*, sweat; 清 *qīng*, clear; 浊 *zhuó*, turbid; 温 *wēn*, warm; 湿 *shī*, dampness

火 (灬) ***huǒ*, fire signific:** 热 *rè*, heat; 燥 *zào*, dryness

月 *ròu* or *rù*, **flesh signific:** 肝 *gān*, liver; 脾 *pí*, spleen; 肾 *shèn*, kidney

耳 *ěr*, **ear signific:** 聋 *lóng*, deaf; 闻 *wén*, listening and smelling; 取 *qǔ*, select; 聚 *jù*, gather

疒 *nè*, **sickbed signific:** 痰 *tán*, phlegm; 病 *bìng*, disease; 疣 *yóu*, wart; 痢 *lì*, dysentery; 痘 *dòu*, pox; 痛 *tòng*, pain

口 *kǒu*, **mouth signific:** 唾 *tuò*, spittle; 古 *gǔ*, ancient; 味 *wèi*, flavor

艹 *cǎo*, **grass signific:** 芍 *sháo*, peony; 艾 *ài*, mugwort, moxa; 芥 *jiè*, mustard plant; 花 *huā*, flower

木 *mù*, **tree signific:** 橡 *xiàng*, oak; 枳 *zhǐ*, bitter orange; 桂 *guì*, cinnamon tree; 林 *lín*, forest; 枝 *zhī*, branch, twig; 根 *gēn*, root

米 *mǐ*, **rice signific:** 精 *jīng*, essence; 粉 *fěn*, powder; 粥 *zhōu*, congee

The significs provide a way of ordering characters in dictionaries so that they can be easily accessed. They are arranged in order of the number of their component strokes, and characters with like significs are arranged together, again, according to the number of their strokes. This method of arranging characters is still used to this day.

Changes in Chinese Script

甲骨文 *jiǎ gǔ wén* Oracle-Bone Inscriptions	金文 *jīn wén* Bronze Script	小篆 *xiǎo zhuàn* Lesser Seal Script	楷书 *kǎi shū* Regular Style

The Chinese script has changed greatly from its beginnings in oracle-bone inscriptions, 甲骨文 *jiǎ gǔ wén*, through the regular style, 楷书 *kǎi shū*, of today. Some of the changes have been due to stylization of graphic elements, while others, perhaps the most important ones, have been due to changes in writing instruments and materials.

During the Yīn-Shāng and Zhōu periods [c. 1600 B.C.E.–c. 771 B.C.E.], bronze casting technology advanced dramatically, and bronze script (金文 *jīn wén*) emerged. Wealthy and noble families possessed large numbers of large bronze vessels, which were the principal symbols of social and economic status.

Every vessel bore inscriptions of characters that had evolved from ancient times. The ancient way of writing these words proved incompatible with the techniques of casting bronze, and so a script was needed that could be cast in bronze artifacts. Thus, as a result of the material properties of working in bronze, certain changes in the form of written characters emerged. Oracle-bone inscriptions were carved on the uneven surfaces of shells and bones. The size and irregular shapes of these bones presented distinct limitations to the writing of characters. Thus as the space available was often small and irregular, the style of writing tended to be small, uneven, and angular. The characters adopted for bronze vessels tended to be much larger and fuller in style than those of the oracle-bone inscriptions. Their component strokes were more smoothly rounded. Like the elegant bronze artifacts themselves, which exhibited a feeling of weight and stability, the inscriptions cast on them were executed in a heavy and stable style.

The era of bronze inscriptions was followed by the Spring and Autumn period [770–475 B.C.E.]. This was a time of decline following the house of Zhōu [c. 1100 B.C.E.–c.771 B.C.E.], which had ruled large portions of ancient China for centuries through a far flung network of feudal fiefdoms. In the Spring and Autumn period, China was divided into many small states and the hundred schools of thought flourished. This led to the period known as the Warring States Period [475–221 B.C.E.]. Kings fought bitterly throughout this period until the leader of one state, Qín, conquered the others and unified China for the first time in its history.

Nevertheless, the unity of the political regime did not bring cultural unity. Each country had its own currency and economic system, as well as its own language, both spoken and written. These various languages are collectively referred to as 古文 *gǔ wén,* or the "ancient language." This is the term used by Xǔ Shèn (许慎 c.58–c.147) who compiled the first known dictionary of Chinese characters, *Shuō Wén Jiě Zì* (说文解字 "Explanation of Simple Graphs and Compound Characters"), when the first Qín emperor issued the decree to unify the written language, currency, and roads. As a result of this process, a new style of script developed. This was the 小篆 *xiǎo zhuàn,* or lesser seal script, which became the official script of the Qín period. It was a simplified derivation of 大篆 *dà zhuàn,* the larger seal inscription, which had been the official script of the Qín state before its ascendancy as the first imperial dynasty. The strokes of lesser seal inscription are smooth and graceful. Each character is set in a rectangular form so that lesser seal script appears more orderly than larger seal script. In Xǔ Shèn's *Shuō Wén Jiě Zì*, all 9,353 entry characters are written in lesser seal script.

At the same time, another step was taken in the development of the written Chinese character. This was the emergence of 隶书 *lì shū*, the clerical script. This style came into existence from the practical consideration that the smooth, curved, and elegantly wavy characters of lesser seal script were impractical for dealing with the heavy daily flow of official documentation. Under pressure to produce extensive daily documentation, lower clerks changed the physical appearance of the official written language in order to make it possible to keep up with the volume of writing to be done. Wherever changes to the character could be made to speed up the writing, whether angling off a round corner or rounding off some more angular places, these changes were implemented. Despite the acceptance and widespread use of clerical script, the two kinds of official style of written Chinese characters coexisted at this time. The lesser seal script was more suited for the elite, and the clerical script, as its name suggests, was for the use of the lower classes.

The emergence of clerical script marked a milestone in the reform of the Chinese character. This change in the history of Chinese written language is referred to as 隶变 *lì biàn,* the clerical style transformation. Scholars normally divide the whole history of the evolution of Chinese characters into two stages: the first stage, known as the ancient stage, is from 甲骨文 *jiǎ gǔ wén*, the oracle-bone script, to the 小篆 *xiǎo zhuàn,* the lesser seal script. This stage spanned more than 1,160 years. The second stage, which started with the emergence of the clerical script and was continued by 楷书 *kǎi shū*, the regular style, and which is known as the latter-day stage, has spanned more than 2,200 years. We can compare the clerical style and modern regular style to find extensive similarities both in structure and style of strokes. The character of clerical script became the core identity of the modern Chinese character. It simplified writing. It laid the basic rules and principles in writing Chinese characters and codified the basic strokes: Dot stroke 点 *diǎn* 丶; horizontal stroke 横 *héng* 一; vertical stroke 竖 *shù* ｜; left-falling stroke 撇 *piě* 丿; right-falling stroke 捺 *nà* 乀; and so forth. The clerical style transformation was a turning point in the development of written Chinese.

The standard style for written Chinese, 楷书 *kǎi shū* or regular style, evolved from the clerical script. There remains some controversy over who invented this style and when it appeared. The general consensus holds that it emerged from the Three Kingdoms period [220 C.E.–265 C.E.]. Some scholars believe this style of writing can be traced back even earlier. Nevertheless, the straight strokes and upright structural characteristics of the regular style secured its position as the standard of written Chinese. It not only pleases visually, but also manifests the central themes of Chinese philosophy such as the importance of uprightness and conformity to cultural norms, which pervade the Chinese worldview. The regular style is both easy to learn and to read; hence it proved to be efficient in communication. It was well developed in the Jìn period [265–420] and came to its height of public acceptance in the Táng [618–916]. To this day it remains a standard style of written Chinese.

Clerical script also gave rise to 草书 *cǎo shū*, grass characters. This way of writing emerged in the Western Han dynasty [206 B.C.E.–25 C.E.]. In this style, all the rules of Chinese handwriting were broken. There is no requirement for regular symmetry, and each character can be proportioned according to one's individual whims. Adjacent characters can be connected or remain distinct. Each stroke can be elongated or shortened, and characters can be either round or square. There are no rules to restrain expression. As a result, this style possesses more artistic value than practical value. It is impractical for ordinary use because it is hard to read; hence, it is confined to calligraphy, which is a major art form in China.

Another style of Chinese writing is known as 行书 *xíng shū,* cursive or running style. It is believed to have originated from the same time period as 楷书 *kǎi shū,* the regular style. It is more fluid and wavy than regular style, but not as unrestrained as the grass characters. It retains the dignity of the regular style, along with far more of its legibility. Thus it proved efficient in daily life and remains prevalent in common use today.

Types of Script

Throughout the course of its evolution, the Chinese script has undergone changes and simplifications. In the modern era, this tendency was expressed by the development of yet another simplification in the written forms of Chinese characters. With the impact of Western culture in the 19th and 20th century, many radical language reformers came to believe that the complexity of the Chinese script was responsible for the low literacy rate in China. Some called for the adoption of phonetic writing and specifically the adoption of the Roman alphabet. With the Communist victory in 1949, prospects of Latinization rose. By the end of the 1950s, however, although a new form of Romanization had been developed (Pīnyīn), simplification of the traditional script had been adopted as a more feasible reform. Though this reform was looked on with scorn in nationalist Táiwān as the destruction of the Chinese heritage, it actually represented a victory for more conservative forces in the mainland who opposed the much more radical proposal to abolish the traditional script and replace it with the alphabet.

篆书〔篆書〕	隶书〔隸書〕	楷书〔楷書〕	草书〔草書〕
zhuàn shū	*lì shū*	*kǎi shū*	*cǎo shū*
Seal Script	Clerical	Regular	Grass Script

In the 1950s, the Chinese government organized the first working group to begin a reformation of the written language. This resulted in the appearance of a new form of Chinese characters known as 简体字 *jiǎn tǐ zì* or simplified script. Of all the various changes and simplifications that the written language has undergone throughout its history, none can equal the scope of this modern development.

The simplified characters come from a variety of new sources, but few are actually new creations. Some are commonly used short-hand forms that had been used for centuries (e.g., 頭 to 头 *tóu*; 當 to 当 *dāng*; 個 to 个 *gè*; 舊 to 旧 *jiù*; 萬 to 万 *wàn*; 禮 to 礼 *lǐ*), or short-hand forms found somewhere in literature (e.g., 陰 to 阴 *yīn*; 陽 to 阳 *yáng*). Others were a reshaping of cursive script (e.g., 為 to 为 *wéi*; 書 to 书 *shū*; 車 to 车 *chē*; 馬 to 马 *mǎ*; 見 to 见 *jiàn*; 門 to 门 *mén*). Still others were archaic forms (e.g., 眾 to 众 *zhòng*; 殺 to 杀 *shā*; 網 to 网 *wǎng*; 從 to 从 *cóng*).

New formations were made by leaving out parts of the character (e.g., 習 to 习 *xí*; 飛 to 飞 *fēi*; 廠 to 厂 *chǎng*), or by simplifying parts after the fashion of cursive script calligraphy (e.g., 幣 to 币 *bì*; 鄧 to 邓 *dèng*; 樹 to 树 *shù*). The most common simplification technique, though, was to replace a complex part of the character with a simple one suggesting the sound (e.g., 藝 to 艺 *yì*; 認 to 认 *rèn*; 態 to 态 *tài*).

Simplification has in some cases entailed elimination of graphic distinction of homophones. 薑 *jiāng* now becomes 姜; 穀 *gǔ* becomes 谷; 乾 *gān* (in some senses) becomes 干; 係 and 繫 *xì* become 系.

While the simplifications have reduced the number of strokes considerably, there is actually no evidence to suggest that the cause of literacy has been served. Literacy is higher in Táiwān, where complex characters are used. Although characters may now be quicker to write, some of them may in fact be harder to learn and recognize than the complex forms.

Even in the People's Republic of China, the complex forms have not completely gone out of use. Historical documents are still often printed in the complex characters. In Chinese medicine, deluxe versions of classics are often produced in complex characters. Given the historical dimension of Chinese medicine, the Chinese student and scholar of Chinese medicine has to be conversant with the complex forms. Since it is quite easy to learn the simplified forms after the complex forms, many Westerners learning Chinese for the purpose of reading medical literature learn the complex form first.

In this book we have presented many ancient forms of the characters discussed, along with both the modern simplified characters and the older complex characters, which are distinguishable from the simplified forms by surrounding brackets. (That is, when you see 阴〔陰〕you will know that the latter character is in the complex form.) These should serve as a comprehensive introduction to the form and meaning of Chinese characters and provide a firm foundation for continued study.

Looking Up Words

Accessing characters in a dictionary takes a little knowledge and practice. In view of the special needs of Chinese medicine, students ideally have to master the differences between accessing simplified and complex characters.

While in English dictionaries alphabetical order is the standard method of arranging entries, indeed in most cases the only way of accessing entries, Chinese dictionaries usually provide more than one means of access. The traditional arrangement of characters in a dictionary was by order of significs. This is the standard arrangement in most modern dictionaries, too. Some bilingual dictionaries published in the PRC (notably *The Pinyin Chinese-English*

Dictionary published by Commercial Press) are arranged in Pīnyīn order. Virtually every Chinese dictionary offers one or more indexes offering another means of access. Some dictionaries will offer an index in which characters are arranged according to the number of strokes composing them. Most dictionaries provide a phonetic index (Pīnyīn in the PRC and Mandarin Phonetic Symbols in Táiwān). And many dictionaries provide a short list of characters whose significs are not obvious.

Accessing by Transcription

Most modern dictionaries have a transcription index. PRC dictionaries regularly contain a Pīnyīn index; some Chinese-English dictionaries have their contents arranged in Pīnyīn order. Táiwān dictionaries often have multiple phonetic indexes, including the Mandarin Phonetic Symbols by which children in Táiwān learn the sounds of Mandarin, but often also the Yale system, and more recently the Pīnyīn system used in the PRC and the West.

For people familiar with Chinese characters and how they are pronounced, consulting a phonetic index is often the simplest way of accessing words in a dictionary. However, accessing by transcription is not so useful a method for the learner who encounters a character he or she has never seen before and has no idea how to read.

Most Chinese characters contain a phonetic element, but most phonetic elements denote several related sounds rather than just one. Sometimes guessing the pronunciation of a character can allow the student to find it quickly, but often it takes several tries, and sometimes it fails to provide access to the character.

Accessing by Significs

It is important to learn this method of accessing characters. Beginning students of Chinese who encounter unfamiliar characters usually have difficulty in guessing their pronunciation and need to access characters by significs. Once students have learned to identify the significs of characters, looking words up by this method is usually quite easy. The significs are arranged in order of the number of their component strokes. Thus, the signific 火 *huǒ*, fire, comes before the signific 黑 *hēi*, black. Characters with like significs are ordered according to the number of additional component strokes. Thus, 燥 *zào*, dryness, with 13 strokes in addition to the fire signific, comes after 灼 *zhuó*, scorch, which only has 3 additional strokes.

For those wishing to master both complex and simplified characters, the difficulty that accessing characters by signific poses is that one character may have a different signific in its complex and simplified forms. For example, the character 下 *xià*, down, which is the same in simplified script as in complex script, has 一 as it signific in complex script and 卜 in simplified script. Furthermore, the set of significs differs from complex to simplified characters. In particular, variant forms of significs in complex characters, such as 月 for 肉, are considered distinct significs in the simplified system.

Of the two systems, the simplified system is probably the easiest to use. One problem with complex characters is that it is not always easy to tell which element of the character is its signific. In the simplification process, character significs in many cases were reassigned to the element of the character that is written first, so that if one is not sure which is the signific, there is a good chance of it being the first element.

Ideally, students should familiarize themselves with all the significs in the Chinese language. However, while some significs, like those of water, wood, grass, and fire, indicate a fundamental element of meaning in a character, other significs are obscure. Many students find that to begin with it is more exciting to get on with the business of learning characters straight away, and learn the significs gradually, starting with the more meaningful ones.

Basic Vocabulary

1. 天 〔天〕 *tiān* Heaven

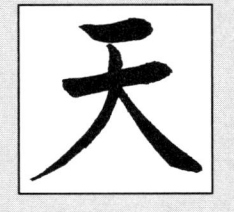

Equivalents
  heaven, celestial

Significs and Stroke Counts
  simplified 大 3 + 1; complex 大 3 + 1

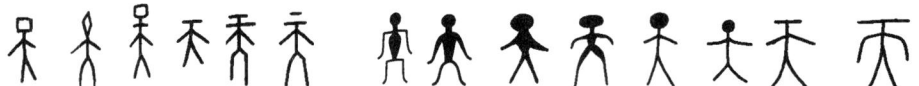

Character Composition

Pictograph. From 一 combined with 大. This character contains 大 *dà*, large or great, which represents a human body with outstretched limbs. It differs by the addition of a mark that emphasizes the head, indicating something large above the human head. Note that 一 is an optional signific for the simplified character.

Explanation

天 *tiān* means sky, heaven; nature; weather. In physical terms, it is the space above the earth's surface, or more loosely what is above human beings. In an abstract sense, it is the highest cosmological principle, that which controls the cosmos.

This character was originally a depiction of a human skull viewed from the front. As time progressed the head was gradually simplified to a short horizontal line indicating the position of the head, i.e., the highest position of the body. Hence, from its original meaning "head" it extended to mean "heaven," "the sky," which occupies the highest position. This meaning was further extended to include "nature," as well as "natural phenomena."

Combinations

天人地	〔天人地〕	*tiān rén dì*	heaven, humankind, and earth
天天	〔天天〕	*tiān tiān*	every day (colloquial)

Stroke Sequence

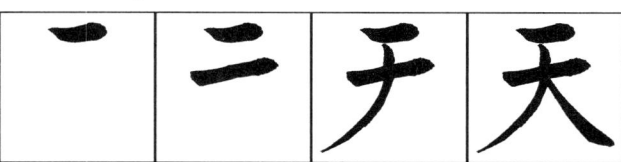

一	二	于	天	天	天	天	天	天
一	二	于	天	天	天	天	天	天
一	二	于	天	天	天	天	天	天

2. 人 〔人〕 *rén* Human

Equivalents
person, human, man

Significs and Stroke Counts
simplified 人 2; complex 人 2

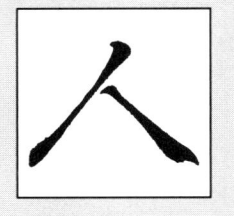

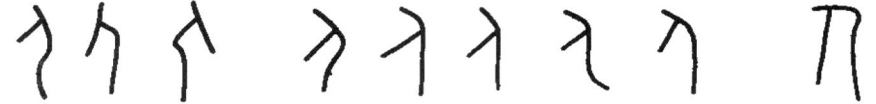

Character Composition
Pictograph of human being in profile.

Explanation
There are many pictographic scripts of 人 *rén* in Chinese, some of them consisting of a picture of a person standing seen from either the front or side view. In others the person is either lying or kneeling down. In some of these versions of the character the figures drawn are of women, children, old people, and so forth. Over time, the side view of a standing man came to be the general character to symbolize the whole human race, mankind, 人 *rén*. Many characters contain the human signific, often in the form 亻. Such characters denote concepts related to human beings, human action, or some similar sense.

Combinations

天人地	〔天人地〕	*tiān rén dì*	heaven, humankind, and earth
大人	〔大人〕	*dà rén*	adult(s)
虛人	〔虛人〕	*xū rén*	vacuous patients
人中	〔人中〕	*rén zhōng*	philtrum; Human Center GV-26

Stroke Sequence

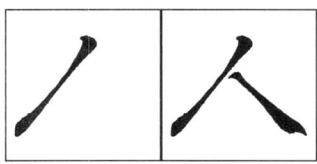

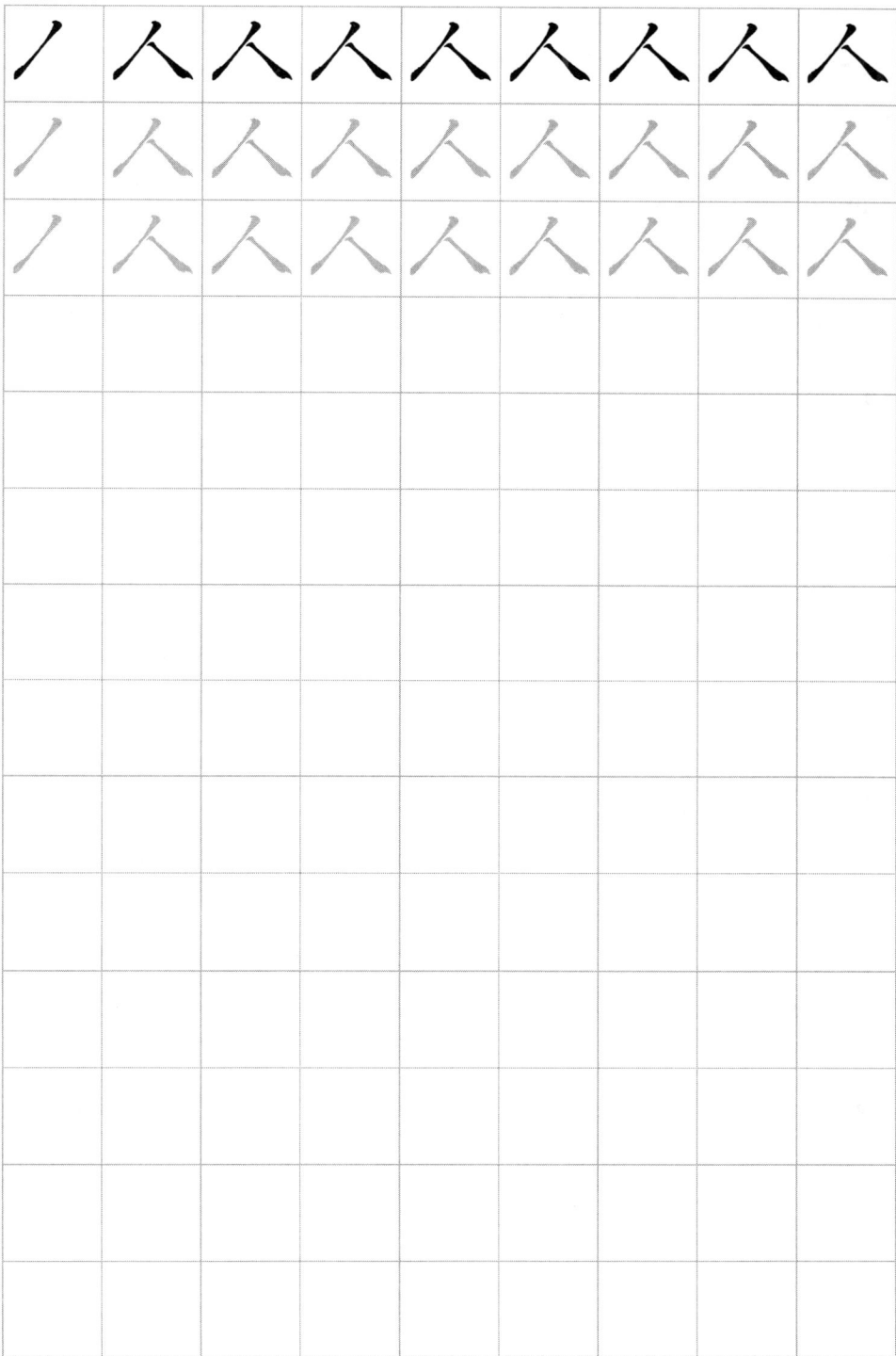

3. 地 〔地〕 *dì* Earth

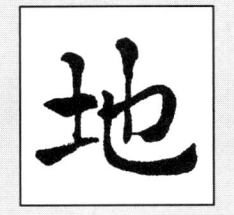

Equivalents
earth

Significs and Stroke Counts
simplified 土 3 + 3; complex 土 3 + 3

Character Composition
Signific-phonetic; earth signific 土 *tǔ* with phonetic 也 *yě*.

Explanation
On the left is the signific component 土 *tǔ*, meaning the earth and, in earlier times, the god of the land. In ancient writing it came to stand for sacrifices to the earth god or altars for such sacrifices. On the right is the phonetic component 也 *yě*. Its ancient pictographic form is a depiction of the female genital organs. Hence, the conjunction of the two components implies the meaning of the "earth," the "receptive power."

Combinations

天人地	〔天人地〕	*tiān rén dì*	heaven, humankind, and earth
天地	〔天地〕	*tiān dì*	heaven and earth
生地黄	〔生地黃〕	*shēng dì huáng*	dried/fresh rehmannia [root]
生地	〔生地〕	*shēng dì*	abbreviation of 生地黄
二地	〔二地〕	*èr dì*	the two rehmannias (i.e., dried/fresh and cooked)

Stroke Sequence

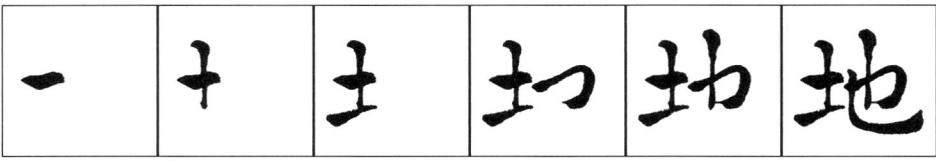

一	十	土	圠	地	地	地	地	地
一	十	土	圠	地	地	地	地	地
一	十	土	圠	地	地	地	地	地

4. 一 〔一〕 yī One

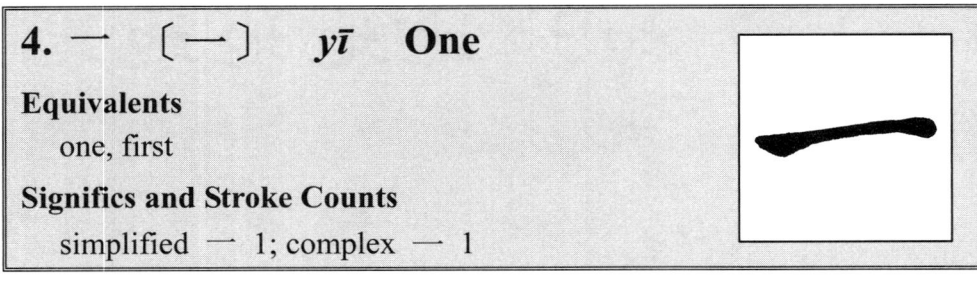

Equivalents
one, first

Significs and Stroke Counts
simplified 一 1; complex 一 1

Character Composition
Ideograph. A single line representing the concept one.

Explanation
In oracle-bone inscriptions, this character was a horizontal line. It may be a figurative denotation of a yarrow stalk, which was used in divination and which conveyed the meaning of oneness and denoted 阳 *yáng*. This drawing of a single horizontal line is a symbol for the abstract mathematical concept of one. Note that the Arabic numeral 1 applies the same representative method, but with a vertical rather than a horizontal line.

Combinations

一阴	〔一陰〕	*yī yīn*	first yīn [channel]
一阳	〔一陽〕	*yī yáng*	first yáng [channel]
一一	〔一一〕	*yī yī*	each; every one
一白二白	〔一白二白〕	*yī bái èr bái*	saururus; Saururi Herba

Stroke Sequence

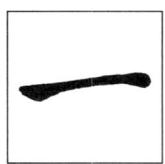

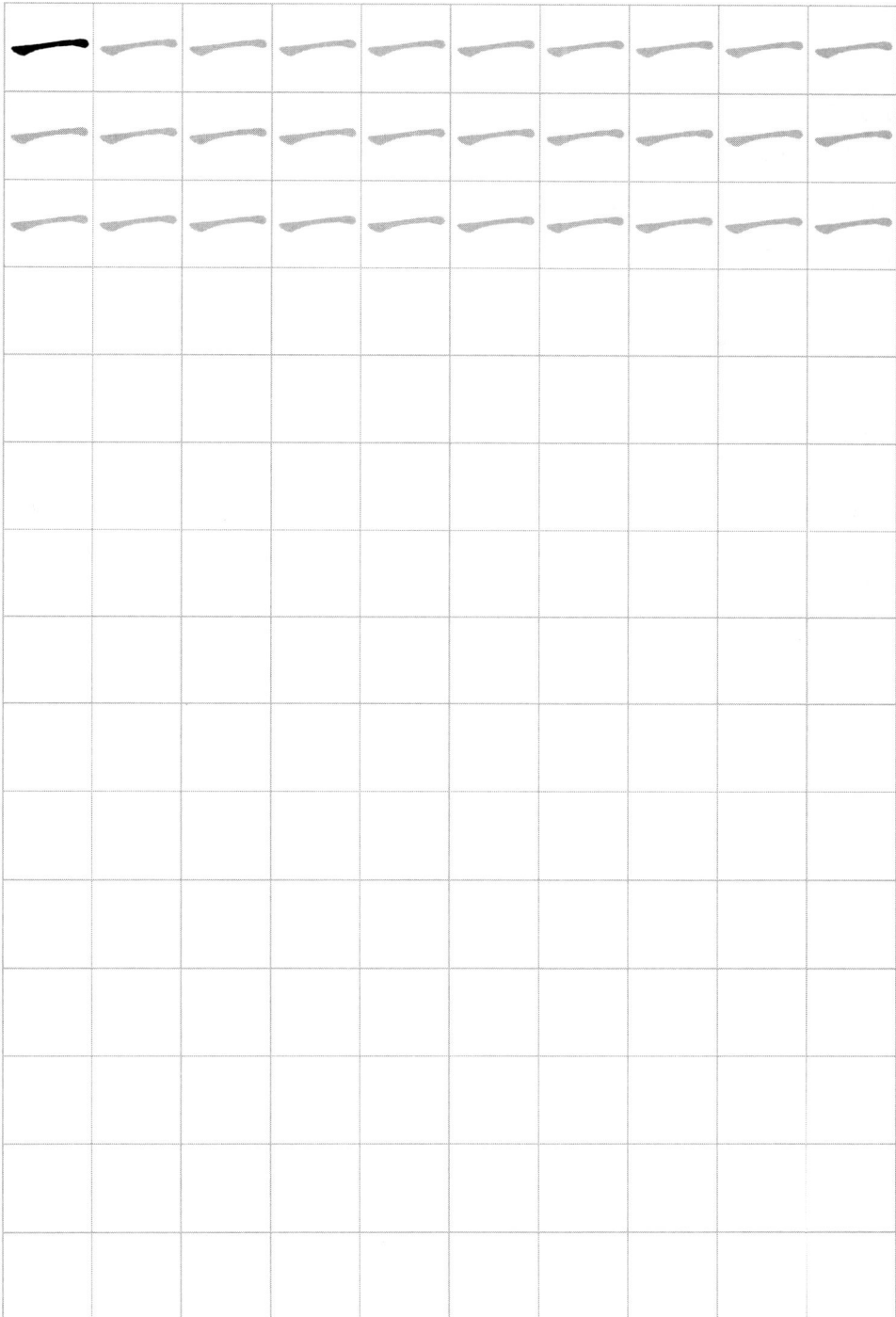

5. 二 〔二〕 èr Two

Equivalents
two, second

Significs and Stroke Counts
simplified 二 2; complex 二 2

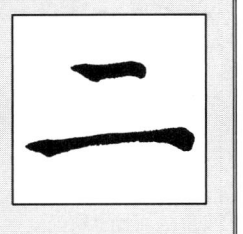

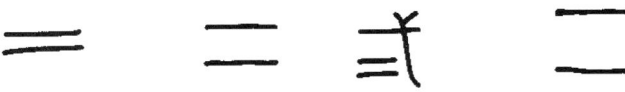

Character Composition
Ideograph. Two lines representing the concept of two.

Explanation
An accumulation of yarrow stalks that symbolizes the number two, the number of the earth, which forms a pair with heaven. The number two is also the symbol for yīn and yáng. Note that the Arabic 2 appears to be similarly formed, but with the lines joined up.

Combinations

二白	〔二白〕	èr bái	Two Whites (point name)
二阳	〔二陽〕	èr yáng	second yáng channel
二阴	〔二陰〕	èr yīn	second yīn channel; two yīn

Stroke Sequence

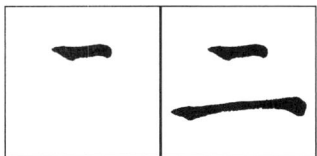

6. 三 〔三〕 *sān* Three

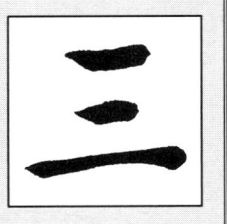

Equivalents
three, third, triple

Significs and Stroke Counts
simplified 一 1 + 2; complex 一 1 + 2

Character Composition
Ideograph. Three lines representing the concept of three.

Explanation
An accumulation of yarrow stalks that symbolizes the number three, the number of heaven, mankind, and earth. Note that the Arabic numeral 3 is similarly formed, but with the lines joined up.

Combinations
三阴	〔三陰〕	*sān yīn*	three yīn [channels]
三阳	〔三陽〕	*sān yáng*	three yáng [channels]

Stroke Sequence

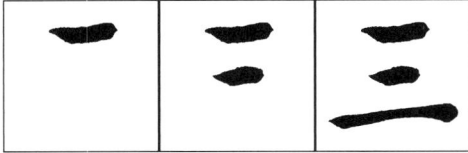

7. 四 〔四〕 *sì* Four

Equivalents
   four, fourth

Significs and Stroke Counts
   simplified ☐ 3 + 2; complex ☐ 3 + 2

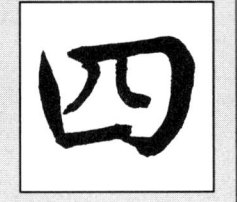

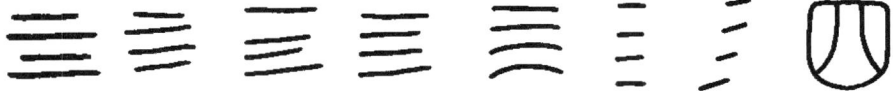

Character Composition
   Ideograph.

Explanation
   None.

Combinations
四白	〔四白〕	*sì bái*	ST-2, Four Whiteness
四大	〔四大〕	*sì dà*	four greatness
四气	〔四氣〕	*sì qì*	four qì

Stroke Sequence

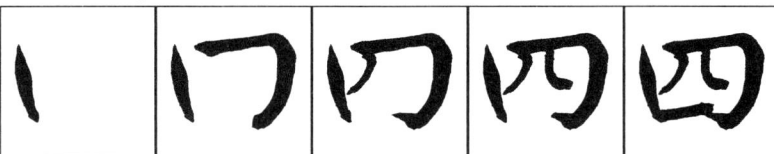

8. 五 〔五〕 *wǔ* Five

Equivalents

five, fifth

Significs and Stroke Counts

simplified 一 1 + 3; complex 二 2 + 2

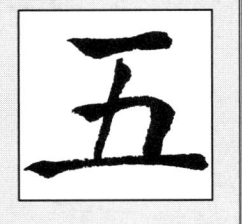

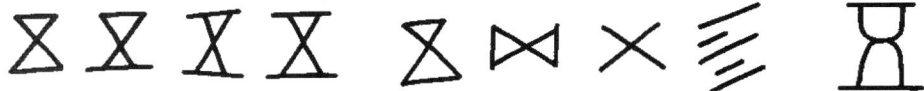

Character Composition

Ideograph. The signific is 二 *èr* in the complex character and 一 *yī* in the simplified.

Explanation

The ancient forms of this character depicted the intersection of heaven and earth, reflecting the special mathematical and metaphorical meanings and the function of the number five in traditional Chinese language and thought. In ancient texts the character was often interchangeable with 午 *wǔ*, probably because of their close resemblance and homophonic relationship.

Combinations

五色	〔五色〕	*wǔ sè*	five colors
五心	〔五心〕	*wǔ xīn*	five hearts
五行	〔五行〕	*wǔ xíng*	five phases
五主	〔五主〕	*wǔ zhǔ*	five governings

Stroke Sequence

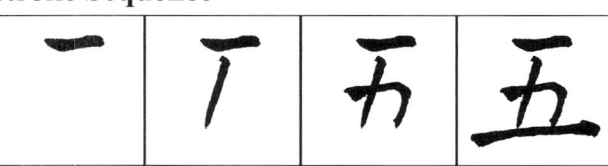

一 丁 㐅 五 五 五 五 五 五 五
一 丁 㐅 五 五 五 五 五 五 五
一 丁 㐅 五 五 五 五 五 五 五

9. 六 〔六〕 *liù* Six

Equivalents

six, sixth

Significs and Stroke Counts

simplified 亠 2 + 2; complex 八 2 + 2

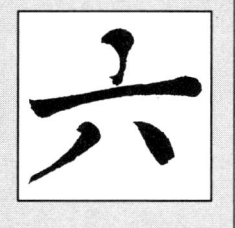

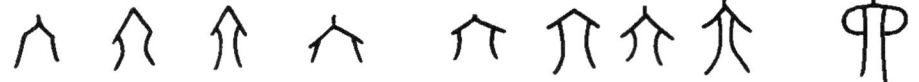

Character Composition

Ideograph.

Explanation

The signific of the complex character is 八 *bā*, eight. The two additional strokes may indicate the number 2, which when deducted from eight leaves six.

Combinations

六腑	〔六腑〕	*liù fǔ*	six bowels
六经	〔六經〕	*liù jīng*	six channels
六气	〔六氣〕	*liù qì*	six qi
六淫	〔六淫〕	*liù yín*	six excesses

Stroke Sequence

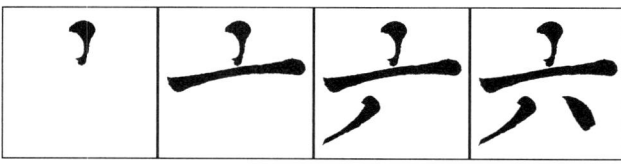

丶 亠 六 六 六 六 六 六 六 六
丶 亠 六 六 六 六 六 六 六 六
丶 亠 六 六 六 六 六 六 六 六

10. 七〔七〕 *qī* Seven

Equivalents
seven, seventh

Significs and Stroke Counts
simplified 一 1 + 1; complex 一 1 + 1

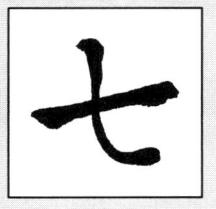

  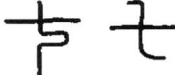

Character Composition
Ideograph.

Explanation
The original meaning of 七 *qī* is cutting, to cut. The 一 *yī* stroke in the middle of ㄴ *yǐn* indicates the action of cutting. The character was borrowed to stand for the mathematical concept of seven.

Combinations

三七	〔三七〕	*sān qī*	notoginseng, Notoginseng Radix
七窍	〔七竅〕	*qī qiào*	seven orifices
七气汤	〔七氣湯〕	*qī qì tāng*	seven qì decoction

Stroke Sequence

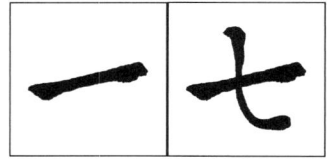

一 七 七 七 七 七 七 七 七 七 七

11. 八 〔八〕 *bā* Eight

Equivalents
eight, eighth

Significs and Stroke Counts
simplified 八 2; complex 八 2

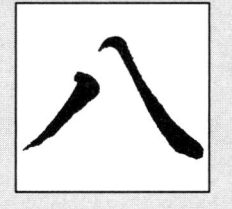

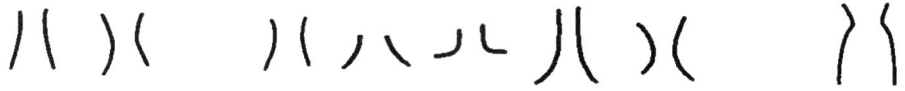

Character Composition
Ideograph.

Explanation
The pictographic form of the character depicts an object split in two halves. The pronunciation also imitates the sound of splitting, and thus many other ancient characters that include the component 八 *bā* relate to the meaning of splitting or division. It is borrowed to symbolize the number eight.

Combinations

八风	〔八風〕	*bā fēng*	Eight Winds (point name)
八邪	〔八邪〕	*bā xié*	Eight Evils (point name)
二十八脉	〔二十八脈〕	*èr shí bā mài*	twenty-eight pulses

Stroke Sequence

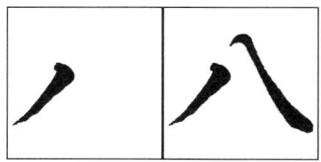

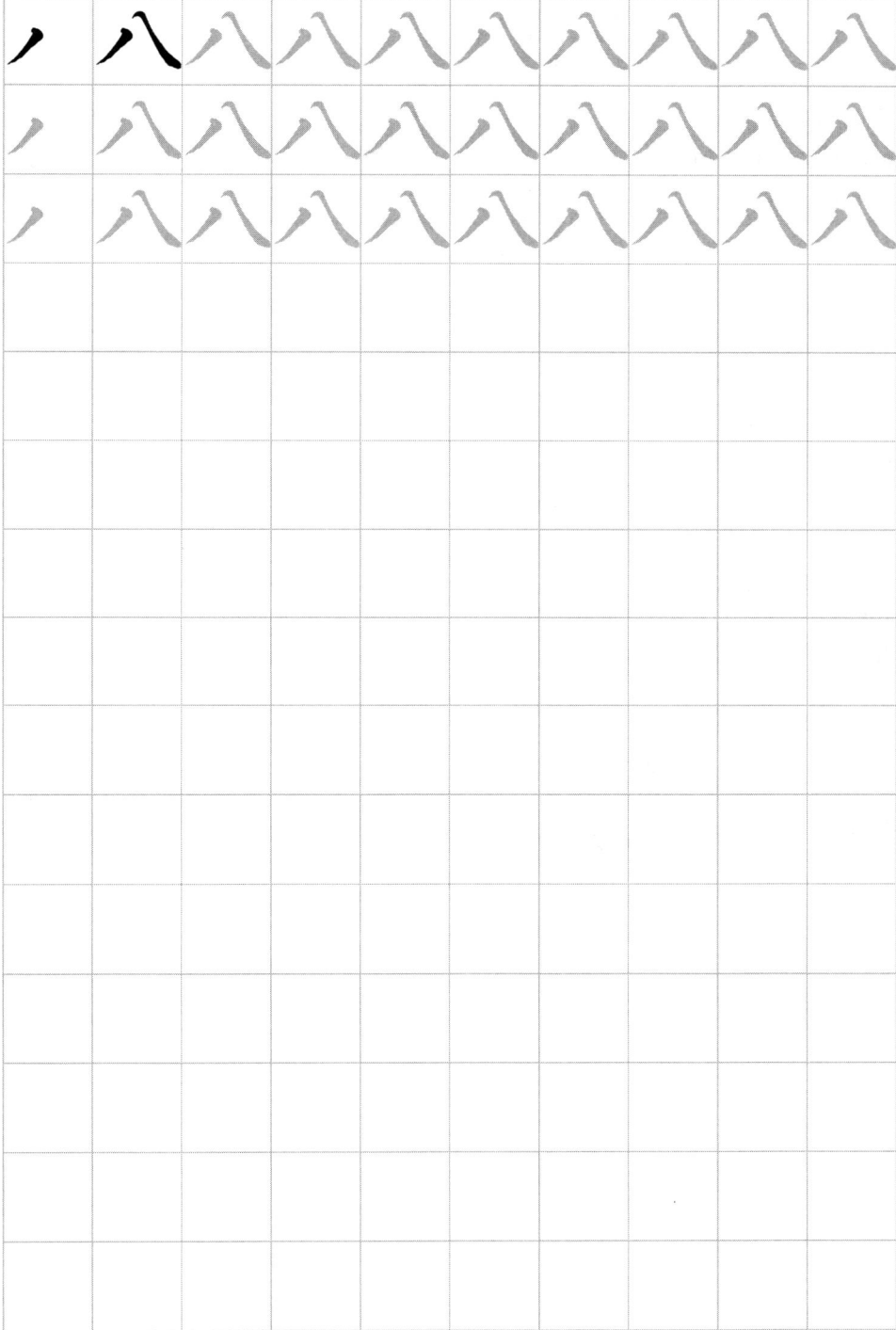

12. 九 〔九〕 *jiŭ* Nine

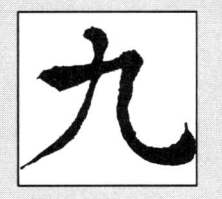

Equivalents
nine, ninth

Significs and Stroke Counts
simplified 乙 1 + 1; complex 乙 1 + 1

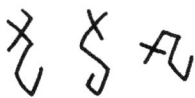 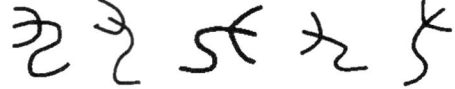

Character Composition
Ideograph.

Explanation
This character is a depiction of a bent elbow. It was used to indicate the number nine. It also came to symbolize things in great amount.

Combinations

九窍	〔九竅〕	*jiŭ qiào*	nine orifices
九克	〔九克〕	*jiŭ kè*	nine grams

Stroke Sequence

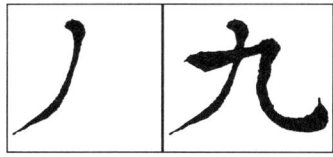

13. 十 〔十〕 shí Ten

Equivalents

ten, tenth

Significs and Stroke Counts

simplified 十 2; complex 十 2

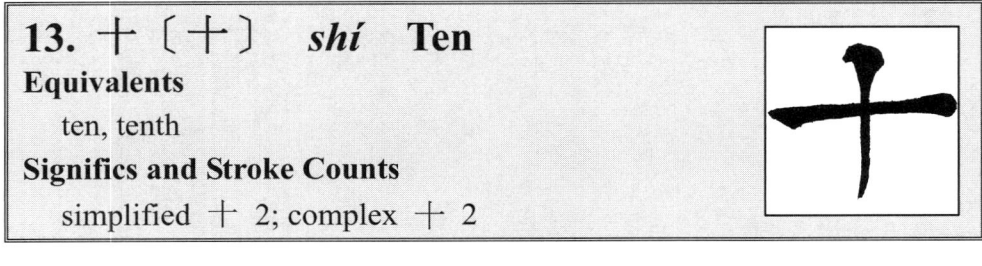

Character Composition

Ideographic. This character was originally written as a vertical line.

Explanation

In ancient forms, the character depicts a knot on a rope, i.e., one unit of counting. In ancient China, there developed a systematic method of denoting numbers. For numbers less than ten, the wooden or yarrow sticks were preferred. Decadal numbers such as twenty and thirty were denoted by tying knots in rope, each knot representing one decadal unit. The symbols in oracle-bone inscriptions were not as obvious. They were vertical lines like hanging rope. Nevertheless, the knots were indicated more clearly in bronze inscriptions, and in some variations the knots were quite visually prominent. The character changed again in the lesser seal script where the dot was elongated to a short horizontal line. The modern character shows the crossing of the horizontal and vertical lines, 十.

Combinations

In Chinese 十一 shí yī, literally "ten [and] one," expresses the idea of eleven; 十二 shí èr, "ten [and] two," expresses the idea of twelve. 二十 èr shí, literally "two tens," is twenty; 三十 sān shí, "three tens," is thirty.

十九	〔十九〕	shí jiǔ	nineteen
二十二	〔二十二〕	èr shi èr	twenty-two
三十三	〔三十三〕	sān shi sān	thirty-three
五十	〔五十〕	wǔ shi	fifty

Stroke Sequence

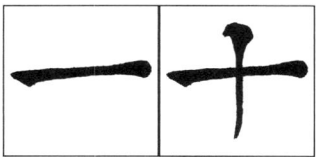

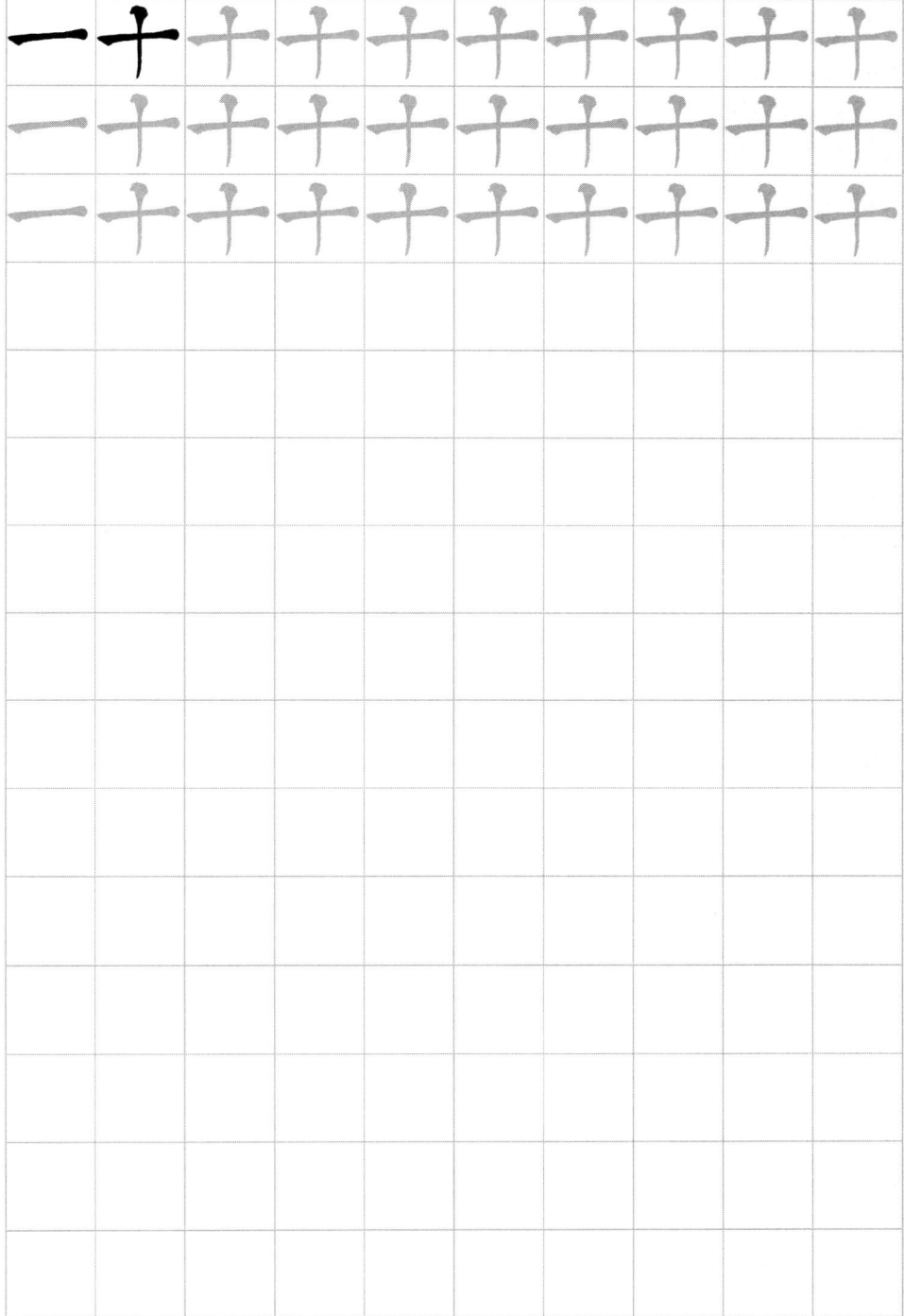

Chinese Medical Characters: Basic Vocabulary

14. 大〔大〕 *dà* Large

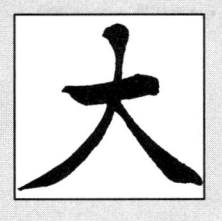

Equivalents

large, great(er), major, adult; also *dài* in 大夫 *dài fu,* doctor, physician

Significs and Stroke Counts

simplified 大 3; complex 大 3

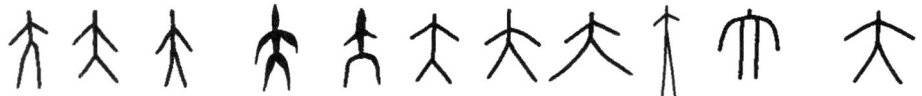

Character Composition

Pictograph. A picture of a man with his arms and legs stretched out to indicate big.

Explanation

This character is a depiction of a standing man with both arms and legs spread apart. The original meaning of 大 *dà* is "adult" or "man of power." This meaning was later extended to mean anything that is larger than other related things, hence, the eventual meaning of "large." When used as a signific in other characters it frequently retains its pictographic meaning.

Combinations

大包	〔大包〕	*dà bāo*	SP-21, Great Embracement
大肠	〔大腸〕	*dà cháng*	large intestine
大风	〔大風〕	*dà fēng*	great wind, leprosy
大汗	〔大汗〕	*dà hàn*	great sweating
大黄	〔大黃〕	*dà huáng*	rhubarb, Rhei Rhizoma
大气	〔大氣〕	*dà qì*	great qi

Stroke Sequence

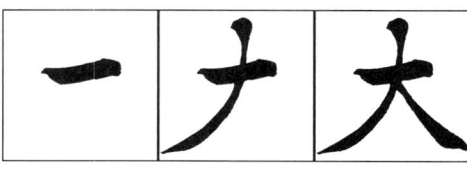

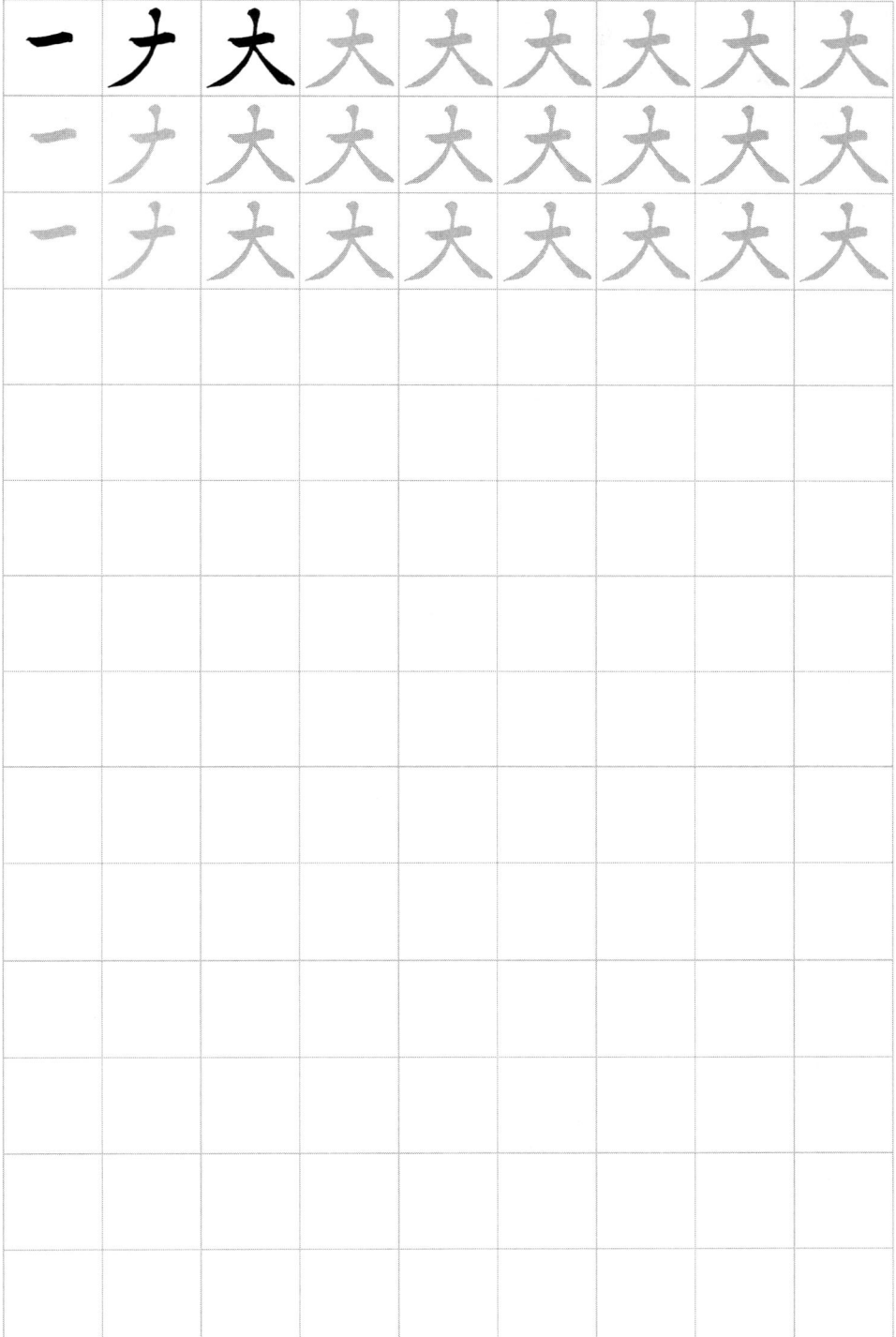

15. 小 〔小〕 *xiǎo* Small

Equivalents
small(er), minor

Significs and Stroke Counts
simplified 小 3; complex 小 3

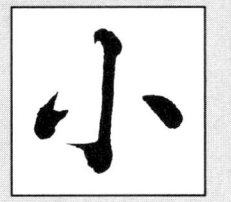

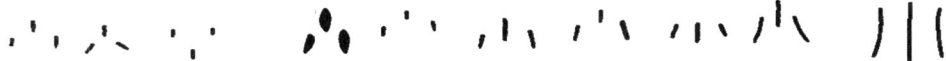

Character Composition
Pictograph. This character was originally written as three dots, indicating small things.

Explanation
The ancient pictograph of 小 *xiǎo* comprises three small dots that symbolize dust, hence, the idea of small. This idea is represented in the modern character by association of 八 *bā,* which in this instance stands for the partition of an object, 亅 *jué,* that is already small by nature. As is often the case in written Chinese, the meaning develops from the reduplication of elements that indicate the overall sense of the word, here, making something that is already small even smaller by dividing it.

In the lesser seal script the middle dot of the ancient character was elongated as if to bisect the whole character into two parts to make it smaller. The meaning of this character extends to include anything smaller or minor.

Combinations
小肠	〔小腸〕	*xiǎo cháng*	small intestine
小脉	〔小脈〕	*xiǎo mài*	small pulse
小水	〔小水〕	*xiǎo shuǐ*	urine

Stroke Sequence

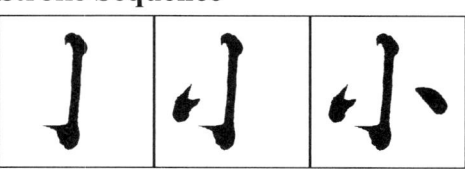

丿	小	小	小	小	小	小	小	小
丿	小	小	小	小	小	小	小	小
丿	小	小	小	小	小	小	小	小
小	腸	小	腸	小	腸	小	腸	
小	脈	脈	脈	脈	脈	脈	脈	脈

16. 中 〔中〕 *zhōng* Center

Equivalents

center, middle; medium; also *zhòng*, strike

Significs and Stroke Counts

simplified | 1 + 3; complex | 1 + 3

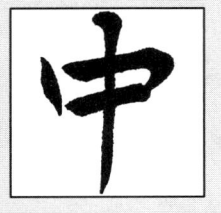

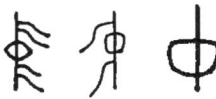 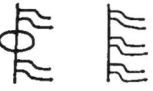 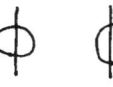

Character Composition

Pictographic representation of a staff with pennants flying in the wind.

Explanation

In ancient China, banners were arrayed on flagpoles and used in identifying states, armies, and groups of people. The number of banners on a single flagpole was never arbitrary or without meaning, but was directly proportional to the owner's power and position. For those standards that contained many banners there was a wooden block positioned at the middle of the flagpole to strengthen the pole. This extra wooden piece was called 中 *zhōng*, and from this sense it came to represent the center because its position was exactly in the middle of the pole. Its meaning also extended to include "medium," "uprightness," and a range of concepts from "central" to "correct." The figurative etymological roots of the word are further reflected in another meaning of 中 *zhōng*, namely to strike or to hit the center, in which case it is read as *zhòng*.

Combinations

人中	〔人中〕	*rén zhōng*	philtrum; GV-26, Human Center
中气	〔中氣〕	*zhōng qì*	center qi
中风	〔中風〕	*zhòng fēng*	wind strike, wind stroke
中人	〔中人〕	*zhòng rén*	strike-on-person
中脏	〔中臟〕	*zhòng zàng*	visceral stroke

Stroke Sequence

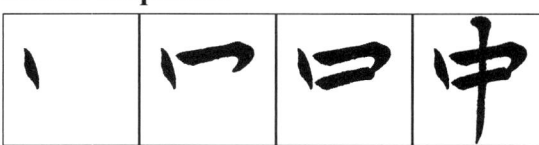

丶 丨 口 中 中 中 中 中 中
丶 丨 口 中 中 中 中 中 中
丶 丨 口 中 中 中 中 中 中

17. 上 〔上〕 *shàng* Up

Equivalents

up, upper, superior, ascend, rise

Significs and Stroke Counts

simplified 卜 2 +1; complex 一 1 + 2

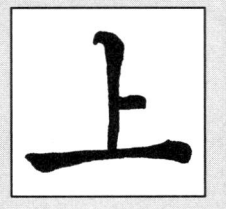

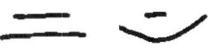  

Character Composition

Ideographic. The horizontal line is a base line, the two strokes above indicate above the base line.

Explanation

The character 上 *shàng* is constructed by the addition of a short horizontal line on a vertical line pointing upward, which indicates that which is above. Hence, the original meaning of 上 *shàng* is that which is up, above. This extends beyond the physical sense to include meanings such as the higher grade, former position in a sequential order, upward motion or action, superior, and ascent.

Compare this to the next character, 下 *xià*, in which the same components are rearranged to indicate below or down.

Combinations

上气	〔上氣〕	*shàng qì*	qì ascent
上窍	〔上竅〕	*shàng qiào*	upper orifices

Stroke Sequence

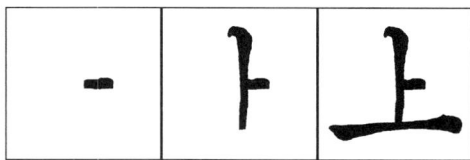

一 卜 上 上 上 上 上 上 上 上

18. 下 〔下〕 *xià* Down

Equivalents
down, lower, precipitate

Significs and Stroke Counts
simplified 一 1 + 2; complex 一 1 + 2

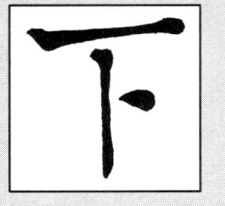

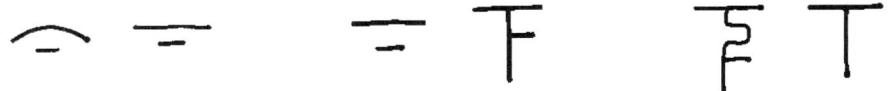

Character Composition
Ideographic.

Explanation
The character 下 *xià* is constructed by the addition of a short horizontal line on the vertical line pointing to the bottom to indicate what is down or below. Hence, the original meaning of 下 *xià* is what is down, below, or beneath. Like 上 *shàng*, its meanings extend beyond the physical sense, to include concepts such as the lower grade, the latter position in a sequential order, downward motion or action, inferior, and descent. Used as an intransitive verb, 下 *xià* means descend; as a transitive verb it means to cause to descend, to precipitate.

Note that some dictionaries use 卜 *bǔ* as the signific for this character.

Combinations
下气	〔下氣〕	*xià qì*	precipitating
下窍	〔下竅〕	*xià qiào*	lower orifices
下阴	〔下陰〕	*xià yīn*	lower yīn
下血	〔下血〕	*xià xuè*	precipitation of blood
上下	〔上下〕	*shàng xià*	above and below; thereabouts

Stroke Sequence

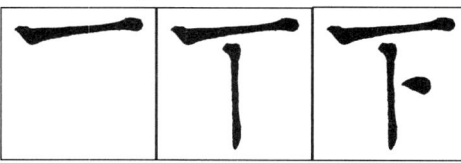

19. 内 〔內〕 *nèi* Internal

Equivalents

internal, inward; also pronounced *nà*, insert

Significs and Stroke Counts

simplified 冂 2 + 2; complex 入 2 + 2

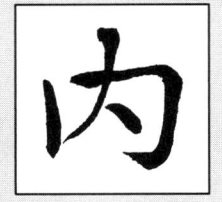

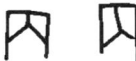   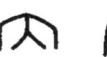

Character Composition

Associative compound.

Explanation

The pictographic form of the character shows a house 冂 *jiōng* and entry 入 *rù* (a variant form of the character 人 *rén*, person). Hence, the meaning of the character is inside, internal, inward.

Combinations

内风	〔內風〕	*nèi fēng*	internal wind
内寒	〔內寒〕	*nèi hán*	internal cold
内火	〔內火〕	*nèi huǒ*	internal fire
内热	〔內熱〕	*nèi rè*	internal heat
内湿	〔內濕〕	*nèi shī*	internal dampness

Stroke Sequence

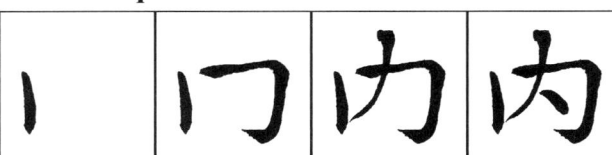

丨	冂	内	内	内	内	内	内	内
丨	冂	内	内	内	内	内	内	内
丨	冂	内	内	内	内	内	内	内

20. 外 〔外〕 *wài* External

Equivalents

external, outward

Significs and Stroke Counts

simplified 夕 3 + 2; complex 夕 3 + 2

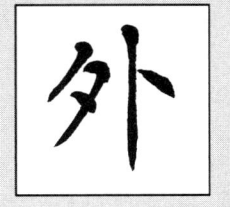

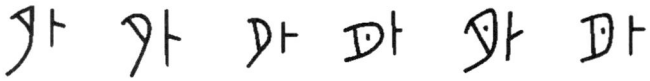

Character Composition

Associative compound.

Explanation

The character is composed of 夕 *xī*, a signific that means moon, and 卜 *bǔ*, a signific that means divination. In ancient China, the divination process consisted of burning both sides of a tortoise shell or other animal bone. The traces on the inner side of the bone after it had been heated were called 内 *nèi* and signified the realm of the self or the host side. The traces on the opposite side were called 外 *wài* and signified the idea of the opponent or the other. Hence, the character 外 *wài* means external, outward.

Combinations

外寒	〔外寒〕	*wài hán*	external cold
外肾	〔外腎〕	*wài shèn*	external kidney
外邪	〔外邪〕	*wài xié*	external evil
外因	〔外因〕	*wài yīn*	external cause

Stroke Sequence

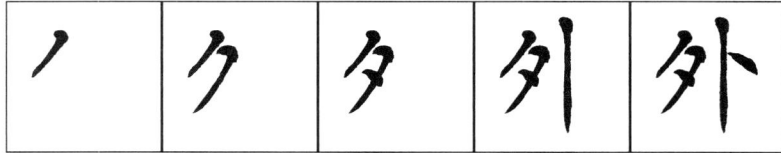

ノ	ク	タ	夕⼁	外	外	外	外	外
ノ	ク	タ	夕⼁	外	外	外	外	外
ノ	ク	タ	夕⼁	外	外	外	外	外

21. 表 〔表〕 *biǎo* Exterior

Equivalents
exterior

Significs and Stroke Counts
simplified 一 1 + 7; complex 衣 6 (4) + 4

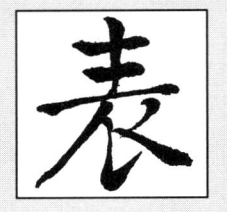

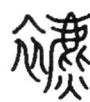

Character Composition

This character is an associative compound that originally depicted a fur coat with the fur on the outside and meant an overcoat. The character was later restyled to incorporate the clothing signific 衣 *yī*.

Explanation

In ancient times, people dressed in animal skins with the fur facing outward. The lesser seal script version of this character consists of 衣 *yī*, clothing, and 毛 *máo*, fur. Thus, the original meaning of the character is "the surface," "the outside," or "the exterior." The meanings of this character also include "signs," "notation," and "norm"; it is used to mean manifestations, i.e., things that manifest outwardly.

Note that the clothing signific of the complex character is split in two, the dot being at the very top of the character—although it is drawn as just part of a longer stroke. (Another character encountered in the terminology of Chinese medicine, 裹 *guǒ*, to swathe, also has its clothing signific split.) Please further note that in certain complex character dictionaries 表 *biǎo* is looked up under the 6-stroke signific 衣 *yī*, yet only 4 strokes from this signific contribute to the overall stroke count.

Combinations

表寒	〔表寒〕	*biǎo hán*	exterior cold
表气	〔表氣〕	*biǎo qì*	exterior qi
表热	〔表熱〕	*biǎo rè*	exterior heat

Stroke Sequence

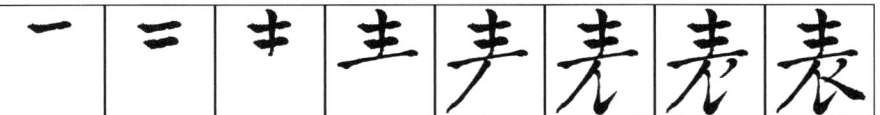

一	二	丰	主	声	表	表	表	表
一	二	丰	主	声	表	表	表	表
一	二	丰	主	声	表	表	表	表
表	表							

22. 里〔裡〕*lǐ* Interior

Equivalents
 interior

Significs and Stroke Counts
 simplified 里 7; complex 衣（衤）6 (5) + 7

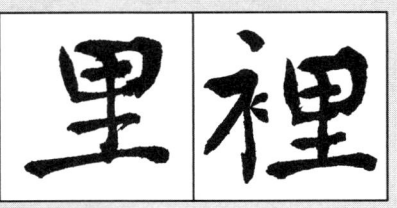

    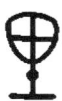

Character Composition

Signific-phonetic compound. The complex character is composed of the clothing signific 衣 *yī* on the left of the phonetic, 里 *lǐ*. The simplified character is simply 里, which is its own signific.

Explanation

In addition to the form of the complex character presented above, 裡 *lǐ*, an alternate form of this character is 裏, and both originally meant the lining of clothing. They both have the clothing signific 衣 *yī*, and the phonetic is 里 *lǐ*. Note that in 裏 the clothing signific 衣 *yī* is split above and below the phonetic.

The character 里 *lǐ* is composed of 田 *tián*, the paddy field, and 土 *tǔ*, the dry land. China has been predominantly an agricultural society since ancient times, and the original meaning of 里 *lǐ* reflects this fact. 里 *lǐ* is the place where people live, i.e., the village. In time this meaning was extended to denote a unit of counting population as well as the basic unit measurement for distance. In ancient China, one 里 *lǐ* was considered to be approximately 500 meters. 里 in these senses is written the same in complex and simplified scripts. In the simplified script, it has replaced 裏 *lǐ* meaning interior. In writings with complex characters, 里 has the meanings explained in this paragraph, but not the meaning "interior."

Combinations

表里	〔表裡〕	*biǎo lǐ*	exterior and interior
里寒	〔裡寒〕	*lǐ hán*	interior cold
里热	〔裡熱〕	*lǐ rè*	interior heat

Stroke Sequence

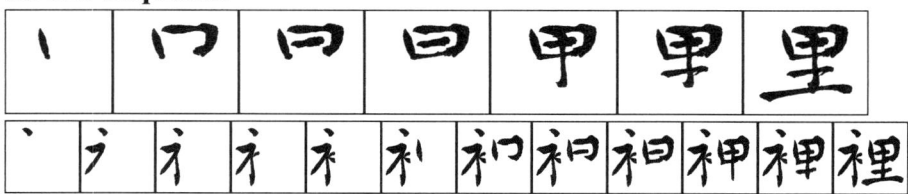

丶	冂	冃	日	甲	甲	里	里	里
丶	冂	冃	日	甲	甲	里	里	里
丶	冂	冃	日	甲	甲	里	里	里

23. 清〔清〕 *qīng* Clear

Equivalents
clear

Significs and Stroke Counts
simplified 氵 3 + 8; complex 水 (氵) 4 (3) + 8

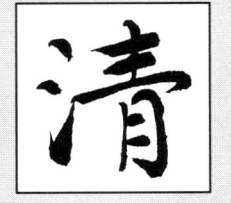

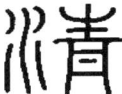

Character Composition

Signific-phonetic compound. On the left is the signific component, 氵 *shuǐ*, water. On the right is the phonetic component, 青 *qīng*.

Explanation

As the phonetic means youth or green-blue, it perhaps gives rise to the meaning of purity through the metaphor of clear blue water.

清 *qīng* is primarily an adjective describing the clear quality of water. In Chinese medicine it is also used as a noun, "the clear," to denote the clean elements of the food and air the body takes in that can be assimilated. It stands in opposition to 浊 *zhuó,* which means foul or waste matter, such as the parts of food that are not absorbed into the body and are passed through the intestines to be eliminated. 清 *qīng* is also a verb, "to clear," in therapeutic terminology. 清热 *qīng rè* means to clear heat, i.e., remove it.

As with many characters that have the three-drop water signific 氵, in certain complex-character dictionaries 清 is to be found grouped under the 4-stroke water signific, 水.

Note that in certain printed fonts, the bottom part of the phonetic has a vertical line instead of a horizontal one, i.e., 清. We have used this variant character in the combinations below, but students do not need to learn to write the character in this way.

Combinations

清肝火	〔清肝火〕	*qīng gān huǒ*	clearing liver fire
清气	〔清氣〕	*qīng qì*	clearing qi
清窍	〔清竅〕	*qīng qiào*	clearing orifices (therapy)
			clear orifice (anatomy)

Stroke Sequence

、	丶	氵	氵一	氵二	沣	浐	清	清	清	清

、	冫	氵	汀	汁	浐	泮	清	清	清
、	冫	氵	汀	汁	浐	泮	清	清	清
、	冫	氵	汀	汁	浐	泮	清	清	清
肝	肝	肝	肝	肝					

漂亮肝

24. 浊〔濁〕 *zhuó* Turbid

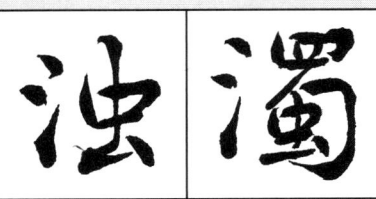

Equivalents
 turbid

Significs and Stroke Counts
 simplified 氵 3 + 6; complex 水（氵） 4 (3) + 13

Character Composition

Signific-phonetic compound. On the left is the water signific 氵 *shuǐ*, on the right is 蜀 *shǔ*, serving as a phonetic, which has been changed to 虫 *chóng*, bug or insect, in the simplified script.

Explanation

The character is constructed with the component 虫 *chóng*, insect or silkworm. 蜀 *shǔ*, which contains 虫 *chóng*, is the ancient name of Sìchuān province in southwest China, the main production area for silk. Hence, the image of worms in the water gives rise to the idea of turbid.

浊 *zhuó* stands in complementary opposition to 清 *qīng,* the preceding character.

Combinations

清浊	〔清濁〕	*qīng zhuó*	the clear and the turbid
浊气	〔濁氣〕	*zhuó qì*	turbid qi
浊窍	〔濁竅〕	*zhuó qiào*	turbid orifices

Stroke Sequence

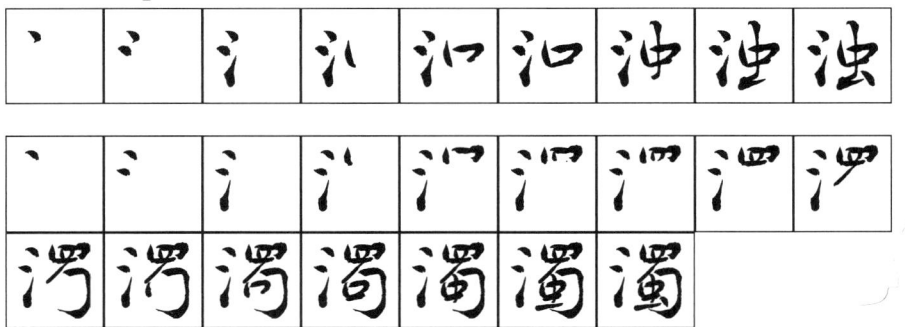

丶	丶	氵	氵	汩	汩	浊	浊	浊
丶	丶	氵	氵	汩	汩	浊	浊	浊
丶	丶	氵	氵	汩	汩	浊	浊	浊
濁	濁							

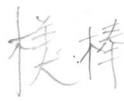

25. 虚〔虛〕 xū Vacuity

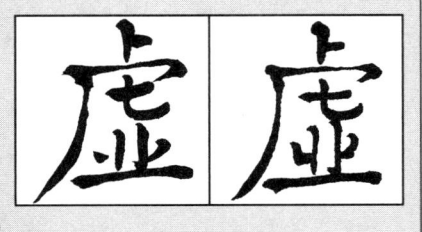

Equivalents

vacuity, vacuous

Significs and Stroke Counts

simplified 虍 6 + 5; complex 虍 6 + 6

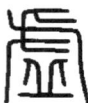

Character Composition

Associative compound. The signific for both simplified and complex characters is 虍 *hū*, meaning a tiger. The lower part of both the simplified and complex is an altered form of the pictograph 丘 *qiū*, a hill.

Explanation

The original meaning of the character was hill or mountain inhabited by tigers or other wild animals. Because a mountain inhabited by wild animals is not inhabited by humans, the meaning was extended to include desertedness or emptiness. The character in its original meaning was changed to 墟 *xū* by the addition of 土 *tǔ*, earth, while the original form came to be used exclusively in the meaning of emptiness.

In medicine, lack of bodily substances, such as qì, blood, yīn, and yáng, are described as 虚 *xū*, vacuities. 虚 *xū* stands in complementary opposition to 实 *shí*, repletion, which is the next character.

Combinations

虚热	〔虛熱〕	*xū rè*	vacuity heat
虚实	〔虛實〕	*xū shí*	vacuity and repletion
上实下虚	〔上實下虛〕	*shàng shí xià xū*	upper-body repletion and lower-body vacuity

Stroke Sequence

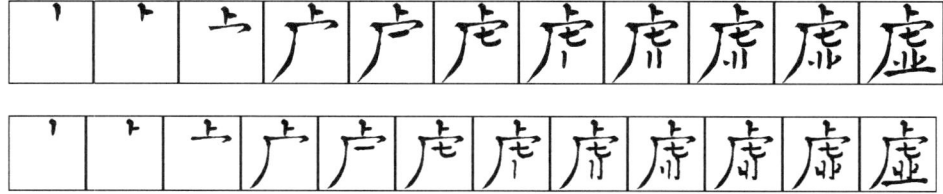

丶 卜 上 广 户 庐 庐 虎 虎 虚 虚

26. 实〔實〕 shí Repletion

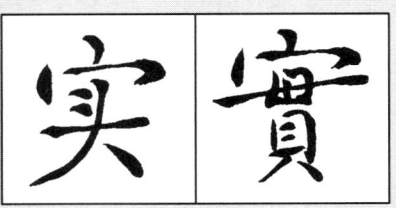

Equivalents

repletion, replete

Significs and Stroke Counts

simplified 宀 3 + 5; complex 宀 3 + 11

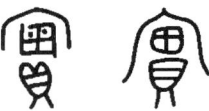

Character Composition

Associative compound. The signific of both the simplified and complex characters is the 宀 *mián*, the roof of a house; on the bottom of the complex character is the component 貫 *guàn*, which means strings of money.

Explanation

The top component is 宀 *mián*, the roof of a house. The upper part of 貫 *guàn*, the lower component of the character, is 毌 *wù*, which depicts a pierced object. The 貝 *bèi*, money, on the bottom symbolizes wealth. Hence, the original meaning of 实 *shí* is wealth, richness. The character extends to mean real, fulfillment, truth, repletion, and replete.

实 *shí* is the opposite of 虚 *xū,* and in the medical context often describes the presence of a disease evil (病邪 *bìng xié*) that is being vigorously fought by the body.

Combinations

实热	〔實熱〕	*shí rè*	repletion heat
虚实	〔虛實〕	*xū shí*	vacuity and repletion
上实下虚	〔上實下虛〕	*shàng shí xià xū*	upper-body repletion and lower-body vacuity

Stroke Sequence

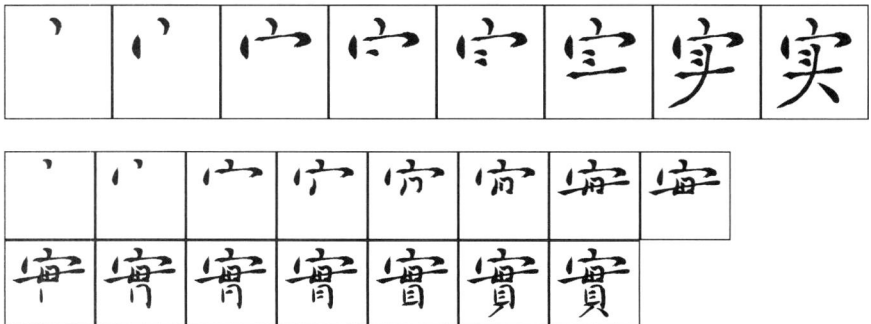

丶	丷	宀	宀	宇	宝	実	实	实	实
丶	丷	宀	宀	宇	宝	実	实	实	实
丶	丷	宀	宀	宇	宝	実	实	实	实

27. 阴〔陰〕*yīn* Yīn

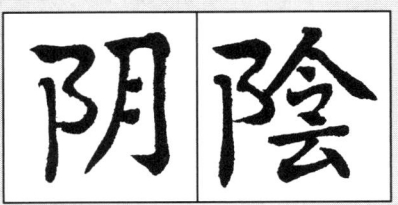

Equivalents

yīn, genital, pudenda, vagina

Significs and Stroke Counts

simplified 阝 2 + 4; complex 阜（阝）8 (3) + 8

Character Composition

Associative compound. Both simplified and complex characters have 阝 *fù*, meaning a mound, as their signific. The right-hand portion of the complex character, 侌 *yīn*, which means shade or shady and is also the phonetic, is more fully described below. In the simplified script, this has been changed to 月 *yuè*, the moon.

Explanation

On the left is the signific component 阝 *fù*, whose earlier pictographic form depicts three steps on a slope. Thus, it came to mean a hill. On the right side of the complex character is 侌 *yīn*, cloudy. It is also composed of two parts: the upper part 今 *jīn*, a phonetic symbol; and the lower part 云 *yún*, cloud. The combination of these two parts results in the meaning of shade or shady. Hence, the character specifically indicates the northern side of the mountain, i.e., the side that is dark and shaded from the sun. This meaning extended figuratively to include a range of objects and phenomena including the female genitals, pudenda, and vagina.

Note that in certain complex character dictionaries this character and the following one are to be found under the 8-stroke signific 阜 *fù*.

Combinations

二阴	〔二陰〕	*èr yīn*	the two yīn
外阴	〔外陰〕	*wài yīn*	external yīn, the pudenda
三阴	〔三陰〕	*sān yīn*	the three yīn [channels]

Stroke Sequence

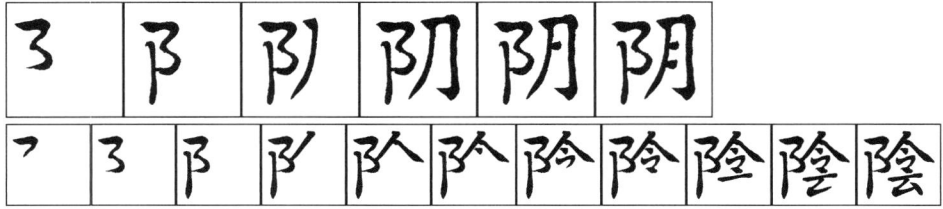

阝 阝 阴 阴 阴 阴 阴 阴 阴 阴

28. 阳〔陽〕 *yáng* Yáng

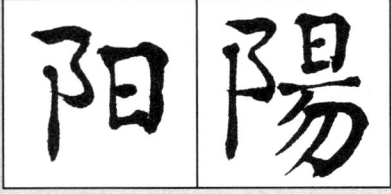

Equivalents
yáng, male

Significs and Stroke Counts
simplified 阝 2 + 4; complex 阜（阝）8 (3) + 9

Character Composition

Signific-phonetic compound. Both simplified and complex characters have 阝 *fù*, meaning a mound, as their signific. The right-hand portion of the complex character is 昜 *yáng*, the phonetic component, which also has the meaning of "brightness." In the simplified form, this has been changed to 日 *rì*, the sun.

Explanation

On the left is the signific component 阝 *fù*, which, just as in the character for 阴 *yīn*, depicts three steps on a steep slope. On the right is 昜 *yáng*, the sun with its rays shining down. The joining of these two characters gives rise to the meaning of 阳 *yáng*: the south, sunny side of a mountain. This meaning extends to include the sun, sunshine, convex, surface, to be exposed outwardly, and male.

Note that the modern expression for sun is no longer 日 *rì*, but 太阳 *tài yáng*, which literally means "the greater yáng" and which is also the name of the acupuncture channels that are associated with the bladder and with the small intestine.

Combinations

阴阳	〔陰陽〕	*yīn yáng*	yīn and yáng; yīn-yáng
三阳	〔三陽〕	*sān yáng*	the three yáng [channels]
脾肾阳虚	〔脾腎陽虛〕	*pí shèn yáng xū*	spleen-kidney yáng vacuity
清阳	〔清陽〕	*qīng yáng*	clear yáng
阳黄	〔陽黃〕	*yáng huáng*	yáng jaundice; yáng yellowing

Stroke Sequence

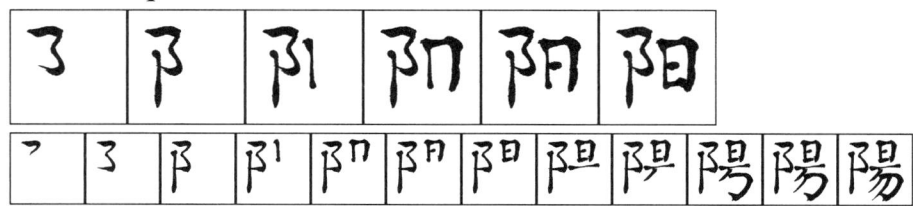

| 了 | 阝 | 阝丨 | 阝冂 | 阝月 | 阝日 | 阝日 | 阝日 | 阝日 | 阝日 |

29. 行﹝行﹞ *xíng* Phase, Move

Equivalents
phase, move

Significs and Stroke Counts
simplified 彳 3 + 3; complex 彳 3 + 3

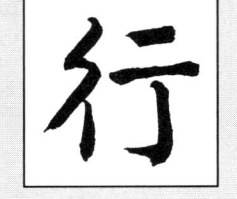

Character Composition
Pictograph. The original character depicted a crossroads to indicate the meaning of to travel or move. The left-hand portion is the signific 彳 *chì*, which originally depicted a T-junction.

Explanation
In both the oracle-bone and bronze inscriptions, the character depicts an intersection of two streets. As the character slowly developed in time, the left side evolved into the shape of a man to indicate people walking on these streets. Hence, the original meaning of 行 *xíng* is street, boulevard, as well as walking, strolling, or movement in general. This meaning extends to column, profession; spreading, transmission, action; phase.

Untrue to etymology, the signific 彳 is often called the "double-person signific" since it looks like 亻 *rén*, a person, with the first stroke duplicated.

Combinations
五行	﹝五行﹞	*wǔ xíng*	five phases
行气	﹝行氣﹞	*xíng qì*	move qì
行气开胃	﹝行氣開胃﹞	*xíng qì kāi wèi*	move qì and open the stomach
温阳行气	﹝溫陽行氣﹞	*wēn yáng xíng qì*	warm yáng and move qì
行水	﹝行水﹞	*xíng shuǐ*	move water
肺主行水	﹝肺主行水﹞	*fèi zhǔ xíng shuǐ*	lung governs the movement of water

Stroke Sequence

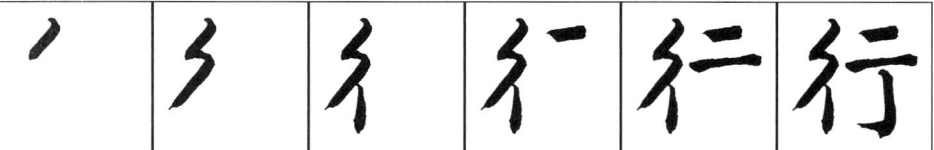

ノ	㇁	彳	彳	行	行	行	行	行	行
ノ	㇁	彳	彳	行	行	行	行	行	行
ノ	㇁	彳	彳	行	行	行	行	行	行

30. 木〔木〕 *mù* Wood

Equivalents

wood

Significs and Stroke Counts

simplified 木 4; complex 木 4

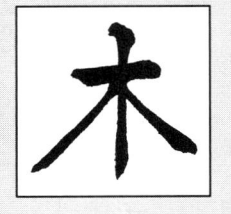

   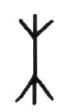 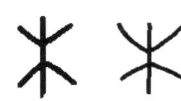 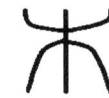

Character Composition

Pictograph of a tree, with its branches and roots.

Explanation

The character 木 *mù* was originally the ordinary word for tree or timber. In modern Chinese, 树 *shù* (which originally meant to plant) has taken over the sense of tree, and 木 *mù* is reserved for the meaning of timber or wood. In the theory of the five phases, 木 *mù* means both tree and wood; it is only by convention that we refer to it as wood in English. This character is also the signific of characters denoting or relating to wood.

In the oracle-bone inscriptions, the character depicts a small tree with its root and branches attached to the stem. Hence, its original meaning is tree. It is a general term for woody plants. It is often used to mean wood, timber, or anything related to or made from wood. Chinese characters constructed with the 木 *mù* component are generally related to wood.

Combinations

木生火	〔木生火〕	*mù shēng huǒ*	wood engenders fire
水生木	〔水生木〕	*shuǐ shēng mù*	water engenders wood

Stroke Sequence

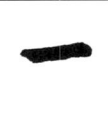 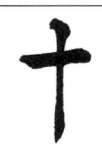 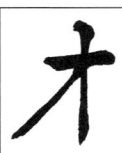 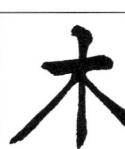

一 十 才 木

31. 火〔火〕 *huǒ* Fire

Equivalents

fire

Significs and Stroke Counts

simplified 火 4; complex 火 4

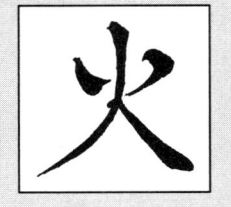

Character Composition

Pictographic representation of flames.

Explanation

In oracle-bone inscriptions, the character depicts a flaming fire. Hence, its original meaning is fire, flame. Chinese characters constructed with the 火 *huǒ* component relate to the idea of fire or flame. This character is also a signific that figures in numerous characters used in Chinese medical terminology. One example is 炎 *yán*, to flame, as in 心火上炎 *xīn huǒ shàng yán*, heart fire flaming upward.

Combinations

火热	〔火熱〕	*huǒ rè*	fire heat
火中	〔火中〕	*huǒ zhòng*	fire stroke
木生火	〔木生火〕	*mù shēng huǒ*	wood engenders fire

Stroke Sequence

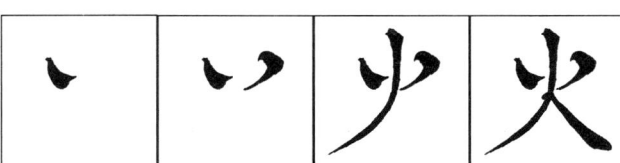

丶	丷	少	火	火	火	火	火	火
丶	丷	少	火	火	火	火	火	火
丶	丷	少	火	火	火	火	火	火

32. 土 〔土〕 *tǔ* Earth (soil)

Equivalents
earth (soil)

Significs and Stroke Counts
simplified 土 3; complex 土 3

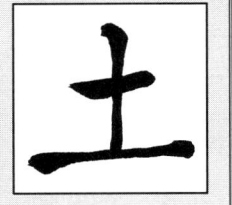

Character Composition

A pictograph of a clod of earth, now represented by the cross, on the ground, represented by the bottom horizontal.

Explanation

In the oracle-bone inscriptions, the character depicts a small mound of earth. Hence, its original meaning is earth, soil, dirt. This meaning later extended to include the land and fields. It was further extended to mean the country or region. Chinese characters constructed with the 土 *tǔ* component relate to the concept of earth or soil.

Combinations

土克水	〔土剋水〕	*tǔ kè shuǐ*	earth restrains water
土生金	〔土生金〕	*tǔ shēng jīn*	earth engenders metal

Stroke Sequence

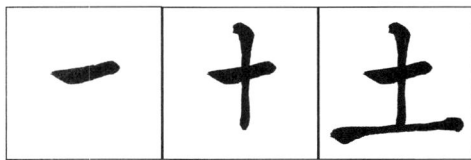

一 十 土 土 土 土 土 土 土
一 十 土 土 土 土 土 土 土
一 十 土 土 土 土 土 土 土

33. 金〔金〕 *jīn* Metal

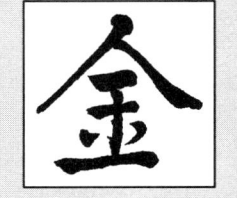

Equivalents

metal

Significs and Stroke Counts

simplified 金 8; complex 金 8

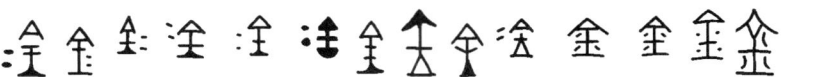

Character Composition

An ideographic representation of a nugget/nuggets of metal dug out of the ground.

Explanation

This character is composed of 今 *jīn* as the phonetic component on top, and 王 *wáng*, a kind of military weapon similar to an ax. The two dots on either side of the bottom of the character represent pieces of ore, which were taken from the earth and refined for making such weapons. Hence, the original meaning of 金 *jīn* is bronze. In general, the character is used to mean metal; later on, it was used almost exclusively for gold. As one kind of currency, the metal gold implies wealth, money, and importance.

This character is also a signific that occurs in characters denoting metals and metal objects. In simplified compound characters, the signific 金 is written as 钅.

Combinations

金生水	〔金生水〕	*jīn shēng shuǐ*	metal engenders water
金门	〔金門〕	*jīn mén*	BL-63, Metal Gate

Stroke Sequence

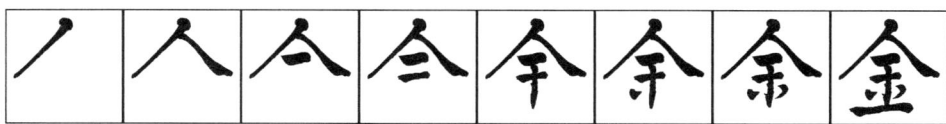

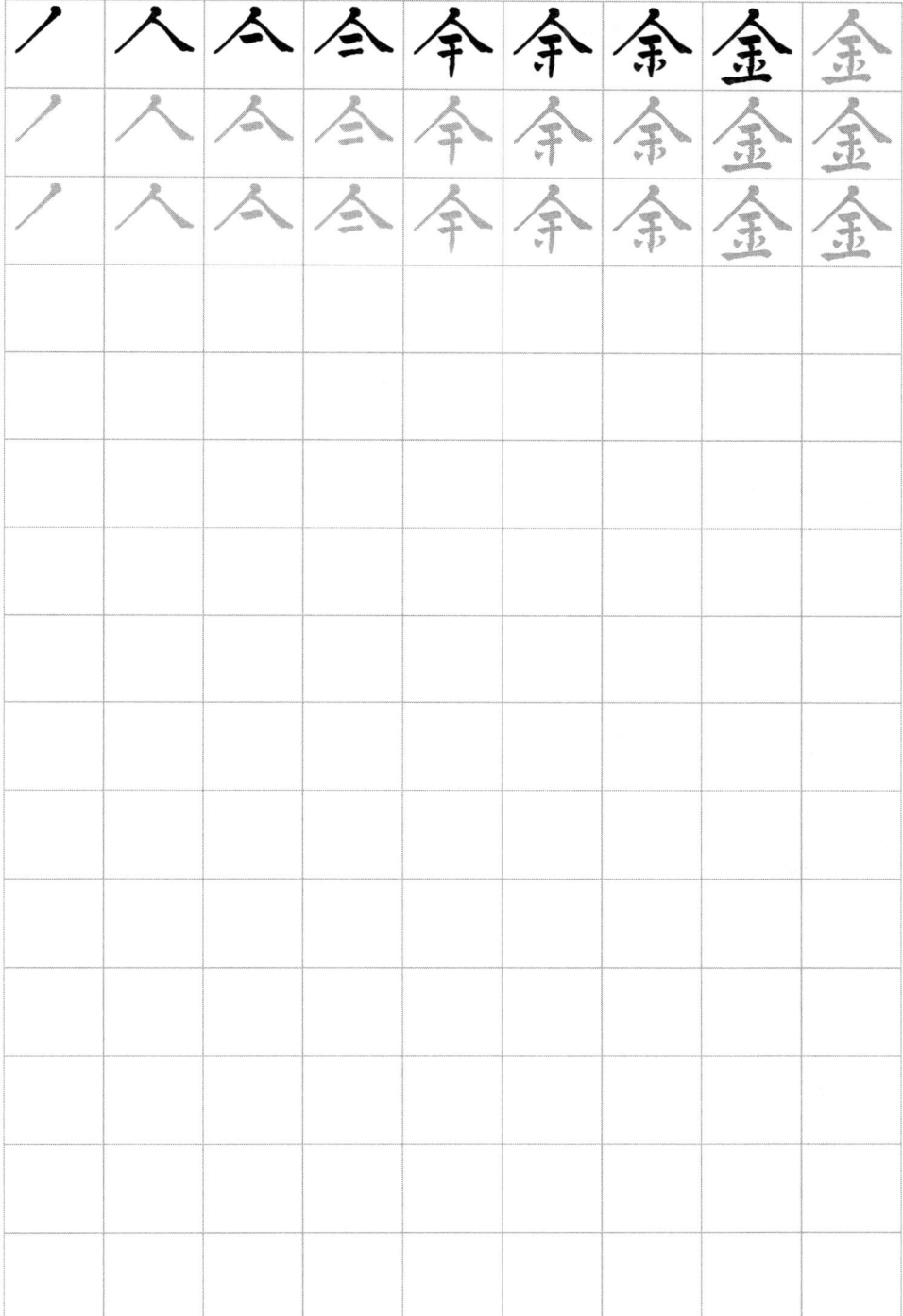

34. 水〔水〕 *shuǐ* Water

Equivalents

water

Significs and Stroke Counts

simplified 水 4; complex 水 4

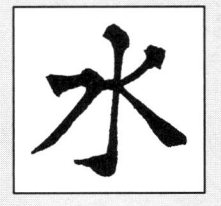

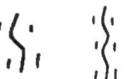 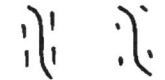 

Character Composition

This character is a pictographic representation of flowing water.

Explanation

The ancient form of the character depicts a current. The center line indicates the main current, and the dots on each side indicate splashes of water. Hence, its original meaning is water. Its extended meaning includes anything in the form of liquid.

This character is also a signific that occurs in characters denoting or relating to fluids. In most of these, it takes on the form of 氵, three drops of water. Eleven of the one hundred characters presented in this book have the water signific: 清 *qīng*, clear; 浊 *zhuó*, turbid; 津 *jīn*, liquid; 液 *yè*, humor; 泪 *lèi*, tears; 汗 *hàn*, sweat; 涕 *tì*, snivel (nasal mucus); 涎 *xián*, drool; 淫 *yín*, excess; 湿 *shī*, dampness; 温 *wēn*, warm.

Combinations

| 水生木 | 〔水生木〕 | *shuǐ shēng mù* | water engenders wood |
| 水气 | 〔水氣〕 | *shuǐ qì* | water qi |

Stroke Sequence

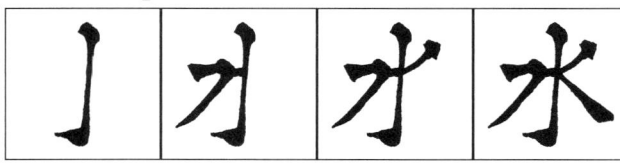

亅 丁 才 水 水 水 水 水 水
亅 丁 才 水 水 水 水 水 水
亅 丁 才 水 水 水 水 水 水

35. 生 〔生〕 *shēng* Engender

Equivalents

engender, arise, vital, reproduce, fresh, raw

Significs and Stroke Counts

simplified 生 5; complex 生 5

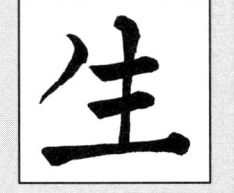

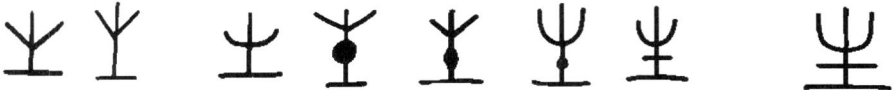

Character Composition

A pictograph of a seed sprouting out of the earth.

Explanation

The oracle-bone form of the character depicts a sprout emerging above the surface of the earth. In the bronze inscription form, a dot is added in the middle of the stem, to indicate the growth or the vitality of the sprout. Hence its original meaning is the growth of plants. Later, the word was extended to meanings such as birth, engender, creation, growth. It is also used to mean aliveness, life, and life span, as well as fresh or raw when used in association with medicinals.

Combinations

木生火	〔木生火〕	*mù shēng huǒ*	wood engenders fire
火生土	〔火生土〕	*huǒ shēng tǔ*	fire engenders earth
土生金	〔土生金〕	*tǔ shēng jīn*	earth engenders metal
金生水	〔金生水〕	*jīn shēng shuǐ*	metal engenders water
水生木	〔水生木〕	*shuǐ shēng mù*	water engenders wood
生地黄	〔生地黃〕	*shēng dì huáng*	raw rehmannia (Rehmanniae Radix Cruda)

Stroke Sequence

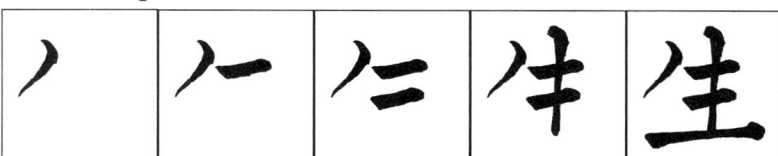

| ノ | ㇓一 | ㇓二 | 牛 | 生 | 生 | 生 | 生 | 生 |

36. 克〔剋〕kè Restrain

Equivalents
restrain; grams

Significs and Stroke Counts
simplified 十 2 + 5; complex 刀 2 + 7

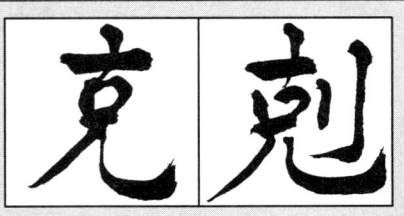

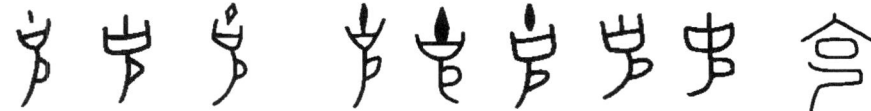

Character Composition

Pictograph. The modern simplified character is a stylized version of a picture of a hooked instrument used to remove the skins from animals. The complex character is often the same as the simplified, but usually a variant form is used that includes the addition of 刂, representing 刀 *dāo*, a knife.

Explanation

The upper part of the character depicts a stone knife and the lower part depicts a skinned animal. The skinning action of the image implies the idea of restraint, i.e., to subdue resistance. Hence the meaning of overcome or restrain.

In modern times this character was borrowed to mean grams, and in this sense it is often seen in recipes for formulas. In complex characters, 克 is the form used for this meaning.

Combinations

生克	〔生剋〕	shēng kè	engendering and restraining
木克土	〔木剋土〕	mù kè tǔ	wood restrains earth
火克金	〔火剋金〕	huǒ kè jīn	fire restrains metal
土克水	〔土剋水〕	tǔ kè shuǐ	earth restrains water
金克木	〔金剋木〕	jīn kè mù	metal restrains wood
水克火	〔水剋火〕	shuǐ kè huǒ	water restrains fire

Stroke Sequence

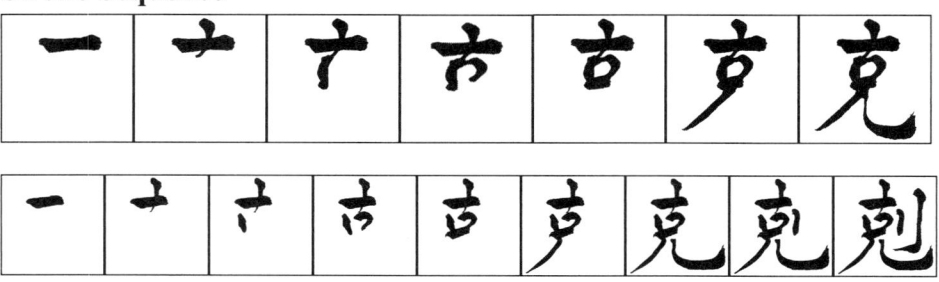

一	十	广	市	古	声	克	克	克
一	十	广	市	古	声	克	克	克
一	十	广	市	古	声	克	克	克

37. 气〔氣〕 *qì* Qì

Equivalents
qì, breath

Significs and Stroke Counts
simplified 气 4; complex 气 4 + 6

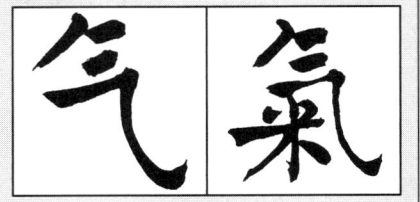

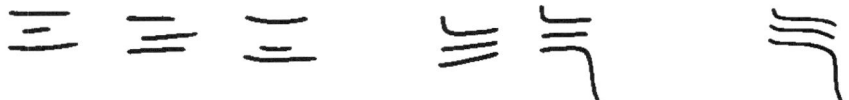

Character Composition

The simplified character is a stylized version of its earliest form, which was a pictographic representation of mist or clouds. The first stroke of the character was a later addition to distinguish it from 三 *sān*, three. A further addition was 米 *mǐ*, grain, symbolizing cooking rice from which fragrant vapor arose.

Explanation

The ancient form of the character depicts a waving cloud. Its extended meaning includes all type of gases as well as many other natural phenomena. 气 *qì* was borrowed by ancient Chinese philosophy to embody certain abstract concepts. From there, the concept of 气 *qì* was also borrowed by all the other disciplines in both ancient sciences and humanities. It is used to describe the condition of the human body both physically and spiritually.

Combinations

阴气	〔陰氣〕	*yīn qì*	yīn qì
阳气	〔陽氣〕	*yáng qì*	yáng qì
四气	〔四氣〕	*sì qì*	the four qì
六气	〔六氣〕	*liù qì*	the six qì
天气	〔天氣〕	*tiān qì*	weather
下气	〔下氣〕	*xià qì*	lower body qì; precipitate qì

Stroke Sequence

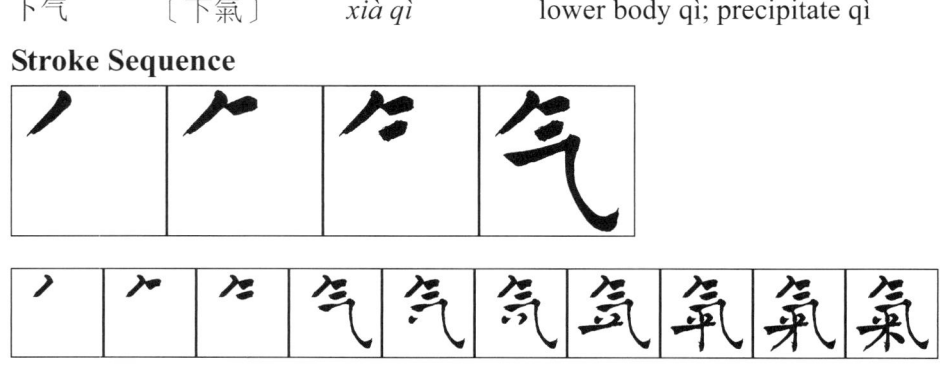

38. 血〔血〕 *xuè* Blood

Equivalents
blood

Significs and Stroke Counts
simplified 血 6; complex 血 6

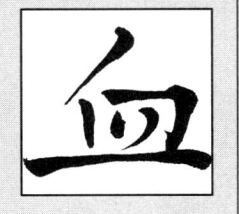

Character Composition

Pictograph. This character depicts a drop of blood dripping into a vessel, 皿 *mǐn*, hence, its original and enduring meaning: blood.

Combinations

阴血	〔陰血〕	*yīn xuè*	yīn blood
气血	〔氣血〕	*qì xuè*	qì and blood
血虚	〔血虛〕	*xuè xū*	blood vacuity
肝血	〔肝血〕	*gān xuè*	liver blood
生血	〔生血〕	*shēng xuè*	engender blood
瘀血	〔瘀血〕	*yū xuè*	blood stasis
下血	〔下血〕	*xià xuè*	precipitation of blood
肝脾血瘀	〔肝脾血瘀〕	*gān pí xuè yū*	liver-spleen blood stasis

Stroke Sequence

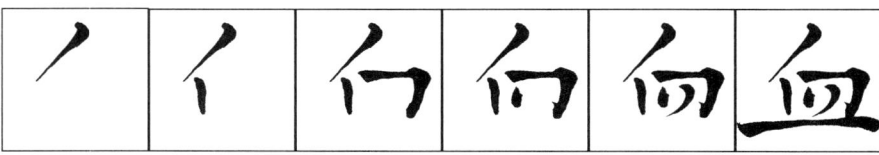

丿 亻 竹 向 向 血 血 血 血

39. 津 〔津〕 *jīn* Liquid

Equivalents

liquid, fluid

Significs and Stroke Counts

simplified 氵 3 + 6; complex 水（氵）4 (3) + 6

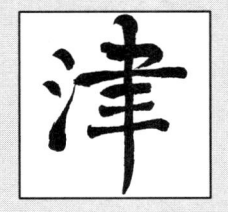

Character Composition

Signific-phonetic compound. On the left is the signific component 氵 *shuǐ*, the water. The original phonetic component on the right was pronounced *jīn*, but it was contracted to 聿 *yù* (a writing brush).

Explanation

This character originally meant, and continues to mean, a place where one can cross a river, a ford. Another meaning is liquid, the sense in which it is used in Chinese medicine.

Combinations

气津	〔氣津〕	*qì jīn*	qì and liquid
津血	〔津血〕	*jīn xuè*	liquid and blood
津气	〔津氣〕	*jīn qì*	liquid and qì
生津	〔生津〕	*shēng jīn*	engender liquid

Stroke Sequence

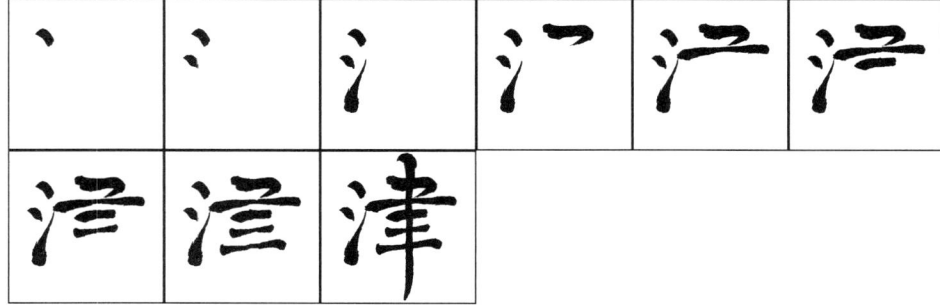

、	丶	氵	氵	汒	汒	泩	津	津
、	丶	氵	氵	汒	汒	泩	津	津
、	丶	氵	氵	汒	汒	泩	津	津

40. 液〔液〕 *yè* **Humor**

Equivalents
humor, fluid

Significs and Stroke Counts
simplified 氵 3 + 8; complex 水（氵）4 (3) + 8

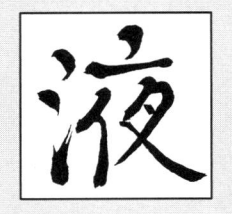

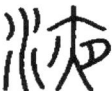

Character Composition

Signific-phonetic compound. On the left is the signific component 氵 *shuǐ*, water. On the right is the phonetic component 夜 *yè*.

Explanation

The phonetic component consists of a person under a roof next to 夕 *xī*, the moon. The synthesis of the two components in this character can give rise to the idea of water retained during the night, hence, humor. While this might be of mnemonic value for learning the character, it is not of clinical relevance.

Combinations

津液	〔津液〕	*jīn yè*	liquid and humor; fluids
肾主水液	〔腎主水液〕	*shèn zhǔ shuǐ yè*	kidney governs water
精液	〔精液〕	*jīng yè*	semen
肠液	〔腸液〕	*cháng yè*	intestinal humor
液燥	〔液燥〕	*yè zào*	dryness of humor
液燥生风	〔液燥生風〕	*yè zào shēng fēng*	dryness of humor engendering wind

Stroke Sequence

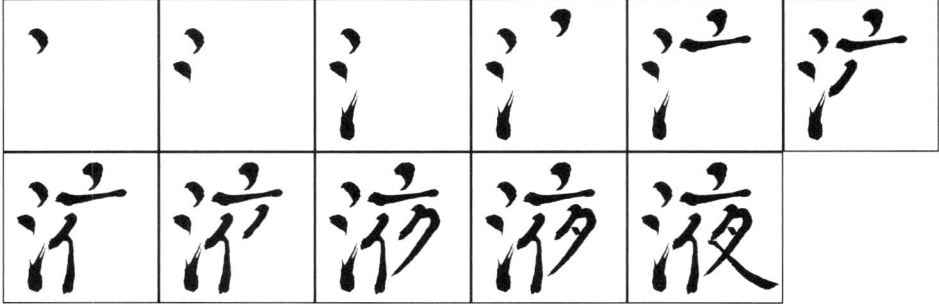

丶	丶	氵	氵	汇	汸	浐	浐	液	液	液
丶	丶	氵	氵	汇	汸	浐	浐	液	液	液
丶	丶	氵	氵	汇	汸	浐	浐	液	液	液

41. 精 〔精〕 *jīng* Essence

Equivalents
essence, semen

Significs and Stroke Counts
simplified 米 6 + 8; complex 米 6 + 8

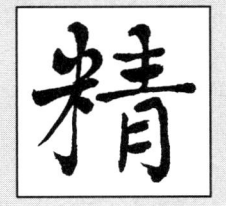

Character Composition

Signific-phonetic compound. On the left is the signific component 米 *mǐ*, rice or kernel of grain. On the right is the phonetic component 青 *qīng*, the color of lush growth, youth.

Explanation

The phonetic could be understood to contribute to the meaning of this character.

As with Character #23 above, certain font faces present the complex character with a variation in the lower part of the phonetic (i.e., in 精, the phonetic is 靑 instead of 青). Students should be able to recognize this variant in reading but do not need to emulate it in writing.

Combinations

精气	〔精氣〕	*jīng qì*	essential qi
精血	〔精血〕	*jīng xuè*	essence-blood
精神	〔精神〕	*jīng shén*	essence-spirit; mind; mental
精寒	〔精寒〕	*jīng hán*	seminal cold
生精	〔生精〕	*shēng jīng*	engender essence
肾精	〔腎精〕	*shèn jīng*	kidney essence

Stroke Sequence

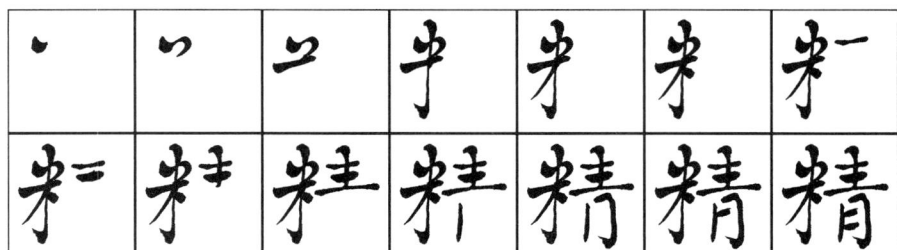

丶	丷	눠	半	半	半	半一	半三	耂	耂	耂	精	精
丶	丷	눠	半	半	半	半一	半三	耂	耂	耂	精	精
丶	丷	눠	半	半	半	半一	半三	耂	耂	耂	精	精

42. 神〔神〕 *shén* Spirit

Equivalents
spirit

Significs and Stroke Counts
simplified 礻 4 + 5; complex 示（礻）5 (4) + 5

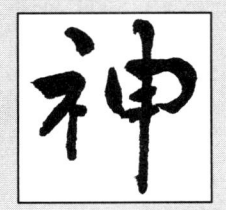

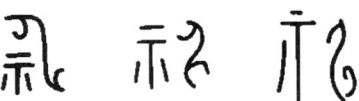

Character Composition

Signific-phonetic compound. On the left is the signific component 示 *shì*, which depicts a totem pole or sacrificial alter; the dots on both sides of the totem pole signify the wine used during sacrificial ceremonies. On the right is the phonetic component 申 *shēn*, which depicts a lightning bolt.

Explanation

There are other characters relating to sacrificial activities that are composed with 示 *shì* as the signific. 申 *shēn* is the prototype of the character 电 *diàn*, lightning, and its meaning was extended to supernatural beings. The combination of these components gives rise to the meaning of spirit, mysteriousness, the supernatural.

In certain complex character dictionaries this character is to be found under the 5-stroke signific 示, even though it is drawn with but 4 strokes.

Combinations

精神	〔精神〕	*jīng shén*	essence-spirit
神气	〔神氣〕	*shén qì*	spirit qi
神门	〔神門〕	*shén mén*	HT-7, Spirit Gate

Stroke Sequence

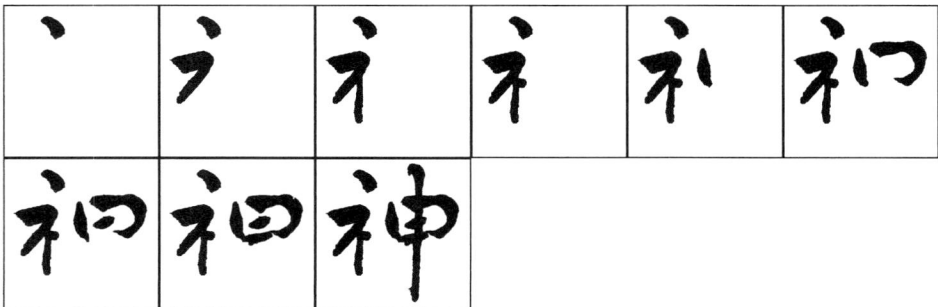

丶 亇 礻 礻 衤 初 初 袒 神
丶 亇 礻 礻 衤 初 初 袒 神
丶 亇 礻 礻 衤 初 初 袒 神

43. 脏〔臟〕 zàng Viscera

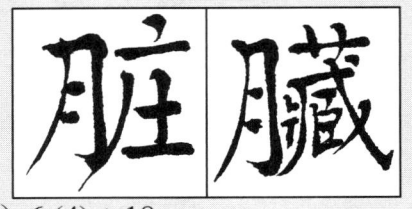

Equivalents

viscus, organ

Significs and Stroke Counts

simplified 月 4 + 6; complex 肉（月）6 (4) + 18

Character Composition

The complex character is a signific-phonetic compound. On the left is the signific component 月 *ròu*, flesh, a variant of 肉. (See the 60th character, 肉, for reference.) On the right is the phonetic component 藏 *cáng*.

Explanation

This phonetic component means conceal, store, or hiding and is composed of grass, 艹 *cǎo*, that covers treasure taken as spoils of war, 臧 *zàng*, on the bottom. Thus, while the character is said to be a signific-phonetic compound according to the traditional classification of characters, it can be thought of as an associative compound.

The components of this character develop the idea of the internal organs that store the essential substances of the body, the viscera. Compare 腑 *fǔ*, the following character. Note that the simplified character obscures the notion of "to store."

Combinations

五脏	〔五臟〕	wǔ zàng	five viscera
脏气	〔臟氣〕	zàng qì	visceral qì
温水脏	〔溫水臟〕	wēn shuǐ zàng	warm the water viscus (the kidney)

Stroke Sequence

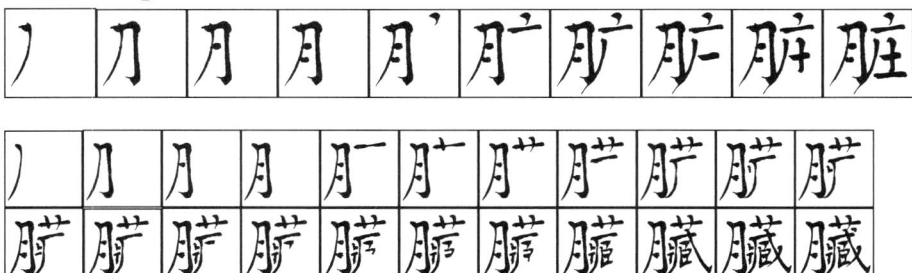

| 丿 | 刀 | 月 | 月 | 月' | 肝 | 肝 | 胪 | 脏 | 脏 |

44. 腑 〔腑〕 *fŭ* Bowels

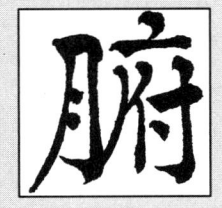

Equivalents
  bowel, organ

Significs and Stroke Counts
  simplified 月 4 + 8; complex 肉（月）6 (4) + 8

Character Composition

Signific-phonetic compound. On the left is the signific component, 月 *roù*, flesh. On the right is the phonetic component, 府 *fŭ*.

Explanation

In this character the phonetic also contributes to the meaning of the character. 府 *fŭ* is an official compound, official archives, official residence, in particular a building where government business was transacted. Thus, the two components give rise to the idea of the organs through which various substances of the body are transmitted, the bowels. Compare 脏 *zàng*.

Combinations

六腑	〔六腑〕	*liù fŭ*	six bowels
脏腑	〔臟腑〕	*zàng fŭ*	viscera and bowels
五脏六腑	〔五臟六腑〕	*wŭ zàng liù fŭ*	five viscera and six bowels

Stroke Sequence

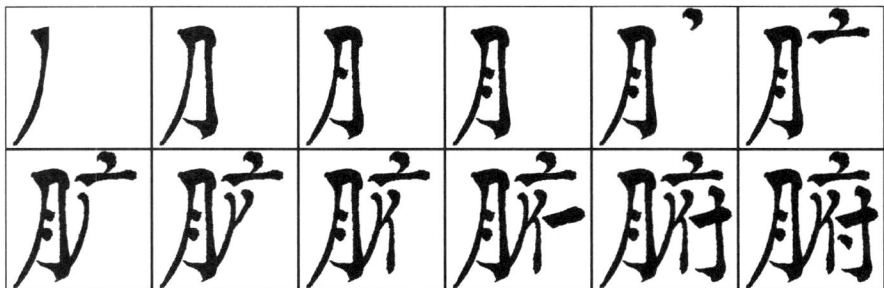

丿	刀	月	月	月'	月⼴	肀	肀	脏	脏	腑	腑
丿	刀	月	月	月'	月⼴	肀	肀	脏	脏	腑	腑
丿	刀	月	月	月'	月⼴	肀	肀	脏	脏	腑	腑

45. 肝〔肝〕 *gān* Liver

Equivalents
liver

Significs and Stroke Counts
simplified 月 4 + 3; complex 肉（月）6 (4) + 3

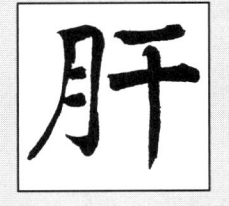

Character Composition

Signific-phonetic compound. On the left is the signific component 月 *ròu*, flesh. On the right is the phonetic component 干 *gān*, which represents the stem or branch of a tree and also a pestle and has the extended meaning of to grind or to destroy.

Explanation

In the past it has been suggested that the element 干 *gān* was chosen because the liver is shaped like stems or branches. While not necessarily historically accurate, this association may be of mnemonic value in memorizing the structure of the character.

Combinations

肝气	〔肝氣〕	*gān qì*	liver qi
肝血	〔肝血〕	*gān xuè*	liver blood
肝阴	〔肝陰〕	*gān yīn*	liver yīn
肝阳	〔肝陽〕	*gān yáng*	liver yáng
肝木	〔肝木〕	*gān mù*	liver-wood
肝火	〔肝火〕	*gān huǒ*	liver fire
肝阴虚	〔肝陰虛〕	*gān yīn xū*	liver yīn vacuity
肝血虚	〔肝血虛〕	*gān xuè xū*	liver blood vacuity

Stroke Sequence

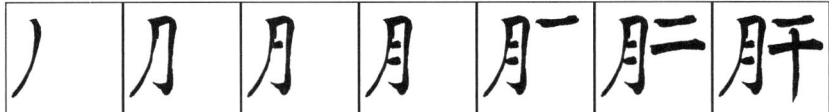

)	刀	月	月	肝	肝	肝	肝	肝
)	刀	月	月	肝	肝	肝	肝	肝
)	刀	月	月	肝	肝	肝	肝	肝

46. 心 〔心〕 *xīn* Heart

Equivalents
heart

Significs and Stroke Counts
simplified 心 4; complex 心 4

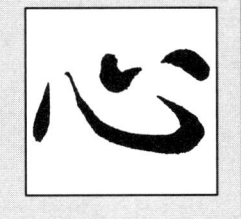

    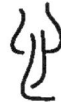   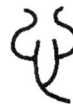

Character Composition

Pictograph. Even in its modern form, this character still recognizably depicts a human or animal heart.

Explanation

In both bronze inscription and lesser seal script, the character follows the shape of the heart. Hence, its original meaning is heart. As the chief internal organ that governs over all others in Chinese medical theory, the heart was considered the source of consciousness. Thus the meaning extends to thoughts, mind, and affection. Since it is located at the center portion of the body, it also comes to mean the center, central. Chinese characters including 心 *xīn* have meanings that relate to thinking, thoughts, ideas, and affection, and often occur in the altered form 忄 *xīn*, as in 情 *qíng,* emotion or affect.

Combinations

心神	〔心神〕	*xīn shén*	heart spirit
心火	〔心火〕	*xīn huǒ*	heart-fire
心气	〔心氣〕	*xīn qì*	heart qì
心血	〔心血〕	*xīn xuè*	heart blood
心阳	〔心陽〕	*xīn yáng*	heart yáng
心阴	〔心陰〕	*xīn yīn*	heart yīn
心气虚	〔心氣虚〕	*xīn qì xū*	heart qì vacuity
心血虚	〔心血虚〕	*xīn xuè xū*	heart blood vacuity
心阴虚	〔心陰虚〕	*xīn yīn xū*	heart yīn vacuity

Stroke Sequence

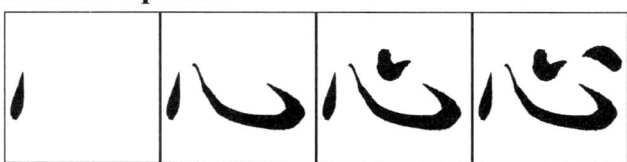

47. 脾 〔脾〕 *pí* Spleen

Equivalents
spleen

Significs and Stroke Counts
simplified 月 4 + 8; complex 肉（月）6 (4) + 8

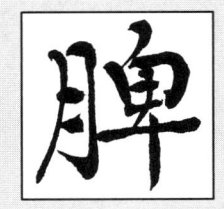

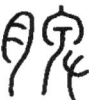

Character Composition

Signific-phonetic compound. On the left is the signific component 月 *roù*, flesh. On the right is the phonetic component 卑 *bēi*.

Explanation

The phonetic 卑 *bēi* is a pictograph of a wine cup with the handle on the left; its extended meaning is common, vulgar, low. Perhaps this element originally was not merely a phonetic, but also a meaning component, reflecting the fact that the spleen is located below the stomach.

Combinations

脾气	〔脾氣〕	*pí qì*	spleen qì
脾土	〔脾土〕	*pí tǔ*	spleen-earth
心脾	〔心脾〕	*xīn pí*	heart and spleen
脾阳虚	〔脾陽虛〕	*pí yáng xū*	spleen yáng vacuity
脾阴虚	〔脾陰虛〕	*pí yīn xū*	spleen yīn vacuity
脾气虚	〔脾氣虛〕	*pí qì xū*	spleen qì vacuity

Stroke Sequence

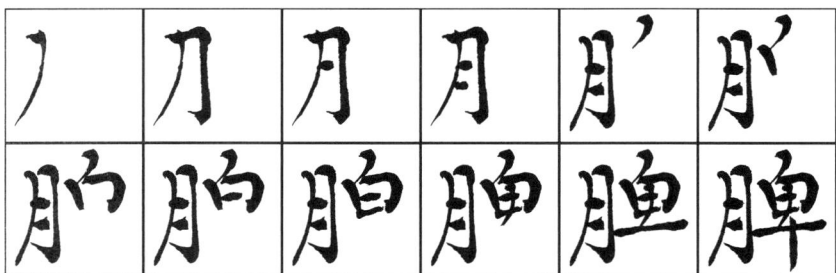

ノ	刀	月	月	月'	𦙶	肑	胎	脾	脾	脾
ノ	ノ	月	月	月'	𦙶	肑	胎	脾	脾	脾
ノ	ノ	月	月	月'	𦙶	肑	胎	脾	脾	脾

48. 肺〔肺〕 *fèi* Lung

Equivalents
lung

Significs and Stroke Counts
simplified 月 4 + 4; complex 肉（月）6 (4) + 5

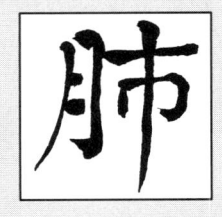

Character Composition

Signific-phonetic compound. On the left is the signific component 月 *ròu*, flesh. On the right is the phonetic component 巿 *fèi*, meaning branching plants that do not stand erect but creep with manifold branches.

In the complex character, the phonetic element is sometimes written as 市 *shì*, market. The etymologically correct form, 巿, was reinstated when the character was simplified in the PRC.

Explanation

The component 巿 has contributed to the meaning of the character, since the lung can be seen as being similar to a plant with manifold branches.

Combinations

肺金	〔肺金〕	*fèi jīn*	lung-metal
肺津	〔肺津〕	*fèi jīn*	lung liquid
肺气虚	〔肺氣虛〕	*fèi qì xū*	lung qì vacuity
肺阴虚	〔肺陰虛〕	*fèi yīn xū*	lung yīn vacuity
肺水	〔肺水〕	*fèi shuǐ*	lung water (lung disease-related water swelling)

Stroke Sequence

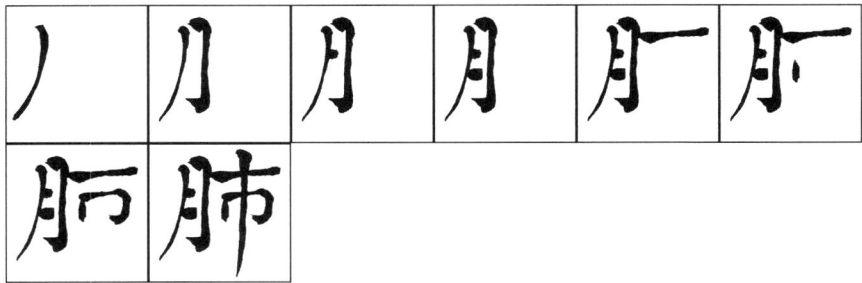

丿 刀 月 月 肀 肝 肺 肺 肺

49. 肾 〔腎〕 *shèn* Kidney

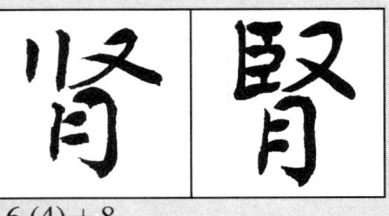

Equivalents
kidney

Significs and Stroke Counts
simplified 月 4 + 4; complex 肉（月）6 (4) + 8

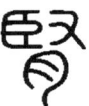

Character Composition

Signific-phonetic compound. The top of the complex character is the phonetic component 臤 *qiān*. Below is the signific component 月 *ròu*, flesh.

Explanation

Although 臤 *qiān* is considered the phonetic component, it can be understood to influence the meaning of this character. It is composed of 臣 *chén*, a servant or an official, controlled by 又 *yòu*, a right hand. Together they mean firm or strong. When this is combined with the flesh signific, the character means strength within the body, the kidney.

Combinations

肾水	〔腎水〕	*shèn shuǐ*	kidney-water
肾阳	〔腎陽〕	*shèn yáng*	kidney yáng
肾阴	〔腎陰〕	*shèn yīn*	kidney yīn
肾精	〔腎精〕	*shèn jīng*	kidney essence
心肾	〔心腎〕	*xīn shèn*	heart and kidney
肝肾	〔肝腎〕	*gān shèn*	liver and kidney
肾气虚	〔腎氣虛〕	*shèn qì xū*	kidney qì vacuity
肾阳虚	〔腎陽虛〕	*shèn yáng xū*	kidney yáng vacuity
肾阴虚	〔腎陰虛〕	*shèn yīn xū*	kidney yīn vacuity

Stroke Sequence

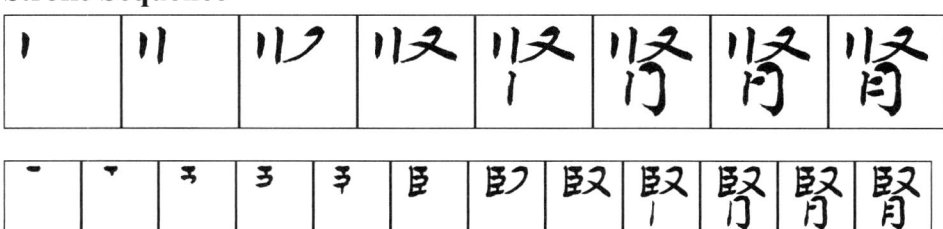

丿	丨丨	丨丿	丨丨又	丨丨又	臤	肾	肾	肾
丿	丨丨	丨丿	丨丨又	丨丨又	臤	肾	肾	肾
丿	丨丨	丨丿	丨丨又	丨丨又	臤	肾	肾	肾

50. 肠〔腸〕 *cháng* Intestine

Equivalents
  intestine

Significs and Stroke Counts
  simplified 月 4 + 3; complex 肉（月）6 (4) + 9

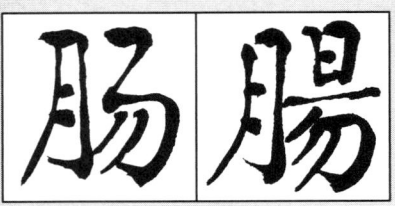

Character Composition

Signific-phonetic compound. On the left is the signific component 月 *ròu*, flesh. On the right is the phonetic component 昜 *yáng*.

Explanation

While in many signific-phonetic characters the phonetic can be understood to influence the overall meaning of the character, in this character we must content ourselves to know that the phonetic only contributes to the pronunciation.

Combinations

小肠	〔小腸〕	*xiǎo cháng*	small intestine
大肠	〔大腸〕	*dà cháng*	large intestine
肠胃湿热	〔腸胃濕熱〕	*cháng wèi shī rè*	gastrointestinal damp-heat
小肠主液	〔小腸主液〕	*xiǎo cháng zhǔ yè*	small intestine governs humor
清大肠邪热	〔清大腸邪熱〕	*qīng dà cháng xié rè*	clear large intestinal evil heat

Stroke Sequence

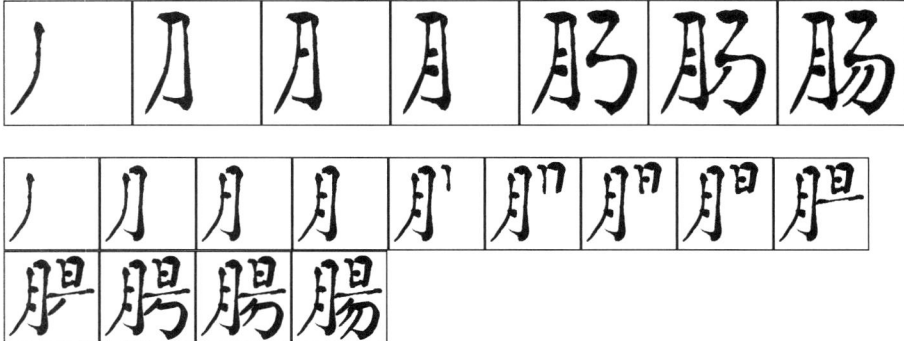

)	刀	月	月	肋	肠	肠	肠	肠
)	刀	月	月	肋	肠	肠	肠	肠
)	刀	月	月	肋	肠	肠	肠	肠

51. 胆〔膽〕 *dǎn* Gallbladder

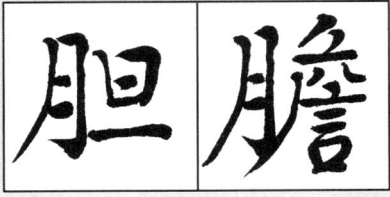

Equivalents
gallbladder

Significs and Stroke Counts
simplified 月 4 + 5; complex 肉（月）6 (4) + 13

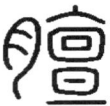

Character Composition

Signific-phonetic compound. On the left is the signific component 月 *ròu*, flesh. On the right of the complex character is the phonetic component 詹 *zhān*.

Explanation

If we examine the phonetic we can conceive how it perhaps affects the meaning of this character. The upper part of the phonetic in the complex character, 厃 *wēi*, depicts a person on a cliff and means danger; the lower part is 言 *yán*, words, and 八 *bā*, to divide or split. If 詹 *zhān* is taken to mean defiant language, this part of the character may possibly reflect the notion of courage, which is an attribute of the gallbladder.

Combinations

肝胆	〔肝膽〕	*gān dǎn*	liver and gallbladder
胆虚	〔膽虛〕	*dǎn xū*	gallbladder vacuity
胆气虚	〔膽氣虛〕	*dǎn qì xū*	gallbladder qì vacuity

Stroke Sequence

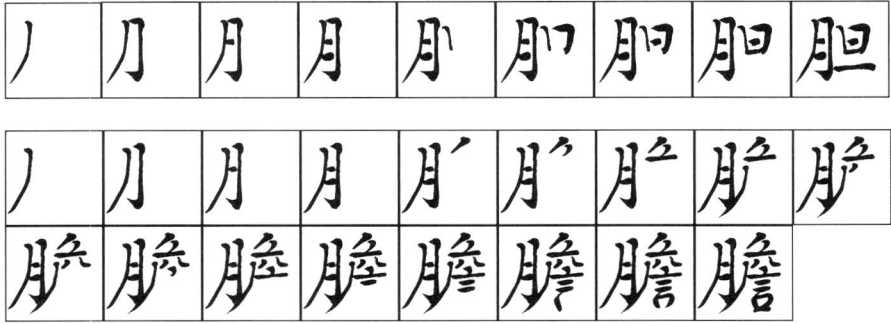

丿 刀 月 月 月 肌 肌 胆 胆

52. 胃〔胃〕 wèi Stomach

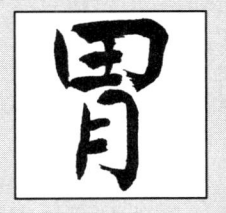

Equivalents
stomach

Significs and Stroke Counts
simplified 月 4 + 5; complex 肉（月）6 (4) + 5

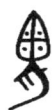 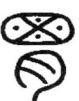

Character Composition

Associative compound. The upper part of the ancient character (see the illustration above) depicts a stomach; the four dots within it represent food in the stomach. The lower part is 月 *roù*, the flesh signific, which imparts the sense of being related to the body and anatomy.

Explanation

The upper part of the modern character is drawn like 田 *tián*, a field; this is a later development from the original ideogram. One might think that the meaning of this character derives from a field related to the body, or the patch of earth within the body, i.e., the stomach. However, historical data indicates this is not the original meaning of the character.

Combinations

胃火	〔胃火〕	wèi huǒ	stomach fire
胃气	〔胃氣〕	wèi qì	stomach qi
胃津	〔胃津〕	wèi jīn	stomach liquid
胃阴	〔胃陰〕	wèi yīn	stomach yin
胃气虚	〔胃氣虛〕	wèi qì xū	stomach qi vacuity
胃阴虚	〔胃陰虛〕	wèi yīn xū	stomach yin vacuity

Stroke Sequence

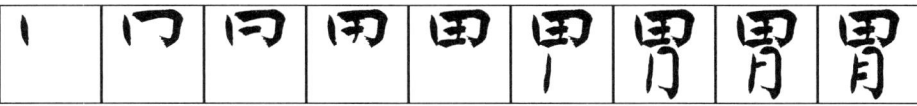

丨	冂	冋	囲	田	甲	胃	胃	胃
丨	冂	冋	囲	田	甲	胃	胃	胃
丨	冂	冋	囲	田	甲	胃	胃	胃

53. 膀〔膀〕 *páng* Bladder

Equivalents

bladder

Significs and Stroke Counts

simplified 月 4 + 10; complex 肉（月）6 (4) + 10

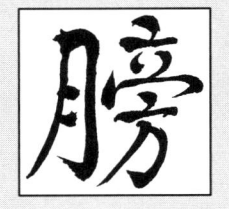

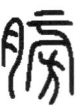 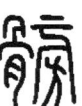

Character Composition

Signific-phonetic compound. On the left is the signific component 月 *ròu*, flesh. On the right is the phonetic component 旁 *páng*.

Explanation

Here is a character where the phonetic appears to act only as a phonetic guide; it seems to make no contribution to or influence on the meaning of the character.

Combinations

膀胱	〔膀胱〕	*páng guāng*	bladder
膀胱湿热	〔膀胱濕熱〕	*páng guāng shī rè*	bladder damp-heat
膀胱气	〔膀胱氣〕	*páng guāng qì*	bladder qi

Stroke Sequence

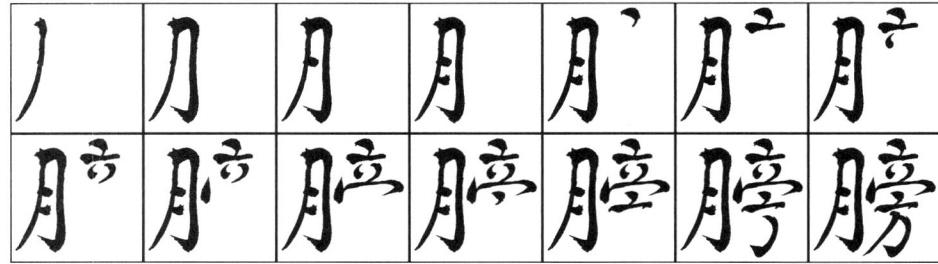

丿 刀 月 月 月` 月⼂ 月⼂ 月ㄍ 月ㄍ 肟 胪 胪 膀 膀

54. 胱〔胱〕 *guāng* Bladder

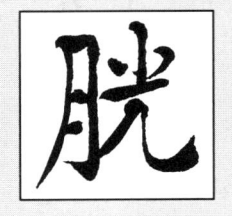

Equivalents

bladder

Significs and Stroke Counts

simplified 月 4 + 6; complex 肉（月）6 (4) + 6

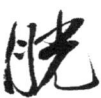

Character Composition

Signific-phonetic compound. On the left is the flesh signific 月 *ròu*; on the right is the phonetic 光 *guāng*.

Explanation

The phonetic is a person 儿 *ér* carrying fire 火 *huò*, meaning light. However, like the preceding character, the phonetic of this character appears to act only as a phonetic guide and does not influence the meaning of the character.

Combinations

膀胱	〔膀胱〕	*páng guāng*	bladder
膀胱经	〔膀胱經〕	*páng guāng jīng*	bladder channel; BL
膀胱虚寒	〔膀胱虛寒〕	*páng guāng xū hán*	bladder vacuity cold

Stroke Sequence

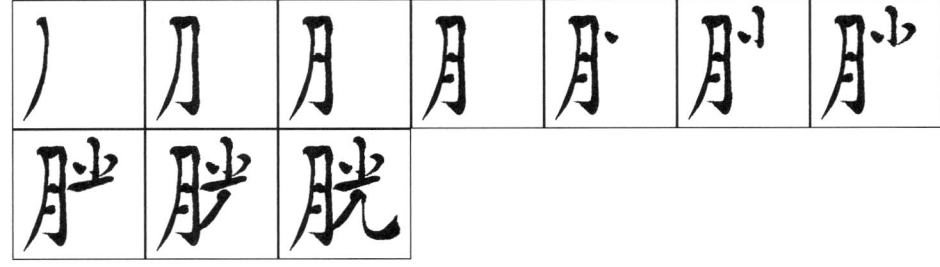

) 刀 月 月 朋 朋 朋 胼 胼 胱

55. 焦〔焦〕 *jiāo* Burn(er)

Equivalents
burn, scorch

Significs and Stroke Counts
simplified 隹 8 + 4; complex 火（灬）4 + 8

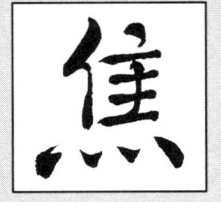

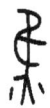

Character Composition

Associative compound. Above is 隹 *zhuī,* a short-tailed bird, and below is 灬 *huǒ,* fire; the whole character thus depicts a bird being roasted. The lower part is the signific of the complex character, and the upper part is the signific of the simplified character.

Explanation

The ancient script of the character depicts bird(s) being grilled over a fire. Hence, its original meaning is "to roast birds." The extended meaning conveys the state of dryness after scorching and also agitation and anxiety. In Chinese medical nomenclature, the figurative sense of "roasting" was adopted to express the notion of the three divisions of the torso understood to be distinct aspects of the body's metabolic processing (or heating and changing) of food and water.

Combinations

三焦	〔三焦〕	*sān jiāo*	triple burner
上焦	〔上焦〕	*shàng jiāo*	upper burner
中焦	〔中焦〕	*zhōng jiāo*	center burner

Stroke Sequence

ノ	イ	亻	亻	仁	佇	住	隹	隹	焦	焦
ノ	イ	亻	亻	仁	佇	住	隹	隹	焦	焦
ノ	イ	亻	亻	仁	佇	住	隹	隹	焦	焦

56. 包 〔包〕 *bāo* Envelop

Equivalents
envelop

Significs and Stroke Counts
simplified 勹 2 + 3; complex 勹 2 + 3

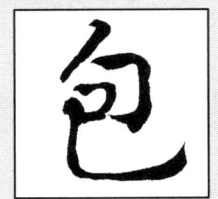

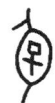

Character Composition

Pictograph. The upper two strokes, 勹 *bāo*, represent the abdomen of a pregnant woman, and the lower part, 巳 *sì*, represents the infant. 勹 *bāo* is the signific, and in itself represents the notion of wrapping. 勹 *bāo* also is the phonetic for this character.

Explanation

The idea of "envelop" is essential to understanding this character. It is the original character for 胞 *bāo*, the placenta. The new character, 胞 *bāo*, composed with the flesh signific, 月 *ròu*, was invented in order to isolate this specific meaning from its extended meanings such as to contain, harbor, or wrap.

Combination

心包	〔心包〕	*xīn bāo*	pericardium
心包经	〔心包經〕	*xīn bāo jīng*	pericardium channel; PC
大包	〔大包〕	*dà bāo*	SP-21; Great Embracement
阴包	〔陰包〕	*yīn bāo*	LV-09; Yin Bladder
心包络	〔心包絡〕	*xīn bāo luò*	pericardium; pericardiac network

Stroke Sequence

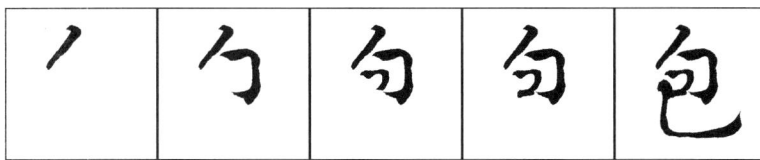

ノ	勹	勺	匀	包	包	包	包	包	包
ノ	勹	勺	匀	包	包	包	包	包	包
ノ	勹	勺	匀	包	包	包	包	包	包

57. 主 〔主〕 *zhǔ* Govern

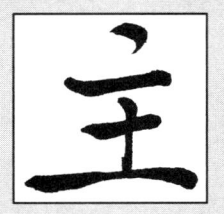

Equivalents
govern(or)

Significs and Stroke Counts
simplified 王 4 + 1; complex 丶 1 + 4

Character Composition

Pictograph. In the bronze inscriptions, the character depicts a burning oil lamp, with the flame 丶 *zhǔ* on the top. In the lesser seal script, the original meaning of 主 *zhǔ* is the wick. In the complex characters, 丶 *zhǔ* came to be the signific; in the simplified characters, 王 *wáng* is the signific—yet certain sources still use 丶 *zhǔ* as the signific.

Explanation

The extended meaning of this character includes host, parent, primary, chief, commander, and govern(or). Later, the character 炷 *zhù* was invented to specifically mean the wick of an oil lamp.

Combinations

心主神	〔心主神〕	*xīn zhǔ shén*	heart governs the spirit
肺主气	〔肺主氣〕	*fèi zhǔ qì*	lung governs qi
主色	〔主色〕	*zhǔ sè*	governing complexion

Stroke Sequence

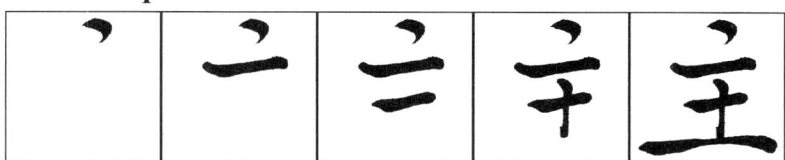

主

58. 筋 〔筋〕 *jīn* Sinew

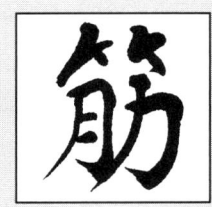

Equivalents

sinew

Significs and Stroke Counts

simplified 竹 6 + 6; complex 竹 6 + 6

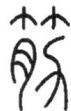

Character Composition

Associative compound. 竹 (⺮) *zhú* bamboo signific on top; 月 *ròu*, flesh, on the left and 力 *lì*, strength, on the right.

Explanation

The strength of the flesh is achieved by the sinews which have the pliable and durable nature of bamboo. The idea of suppleness and flexibility combine to form the idea of sinew, tendon.

Combinations

肝主筋	〔肝主筋〕	*gān zhǔ jīn*	the liver governs the sinews
筋脉	〔筋脈〕	*jīn mài*	sinew vessel
筋骨	〔筋骨〕	*jīn gǔ*	sinew and bone
筋络	〔筋絡〕	*jīn luò*	sinew network vessels
筋肉	〔筋肉〕	*jīn ròu*	sinew and flesh
筋寒	〔筋寒〕	*jīn hán*	cold sinews

Stroke Sequence

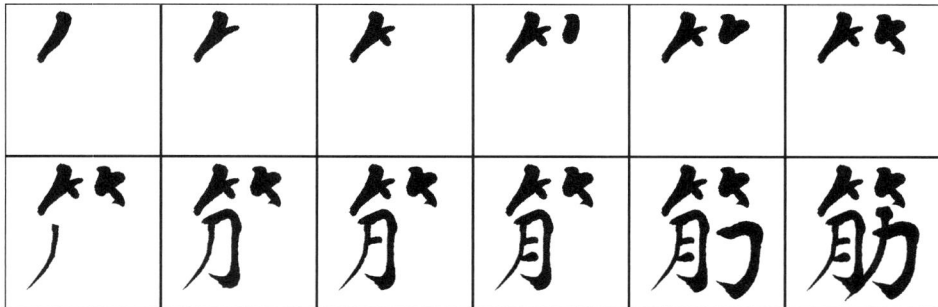

ノ	𠂉	𠂉	𠂉	竹	竹	𥫗	分	笂	笃	筋	筋
ノ	𠂉	𠂉	𠂉	竹	竹	𥫗	分	笂	笃	筋	筋
ノ	𠂉	𠂉	𠂉	竹	竹	𥫗	分	笂	笃	筋	筋

59. 脉〔脈〕*mài* Vessel, Pulse

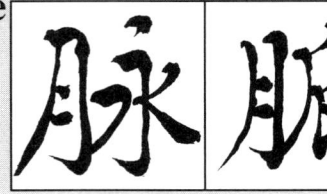

Equivalents
vessel, pulse

Significs and Stroke Counts
simplified 月 4 + 5; complex 肉（月）6 (4) + 6

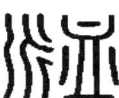 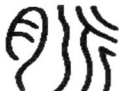

Character Composition

Signific-phonetic compound. On the left is the signific component 月 *ròu*, flesh, on the right is the phonetic.

Explanation

The phonetic component clearly contributes to the meaning of this character, for it is a pictograph that represents a tributary joining the main stream. It is also the reverse of the character 永 *yǒng*, which means the tributaries of a river. An alternative interpretation of this pictographic could be a person swimming in the current. In sum, the interpretation of the phonetic has stabilized around the idea of the tributaries of a main river. Taken as a metaphor, the idea of the character is "vessel" and "pulse" when it is projected onto the physical body, here by the presence of the flesh signific.

Combinations

心主脉	〔心主脈〕	*xīn zhǔ mài*	the heart governs the vessels
脉气	〔脈氣〕	*mài qì*	vessel qi
脉口	〔脈口〕	*mài kǒu*	vessel opening

Stroke Sequence

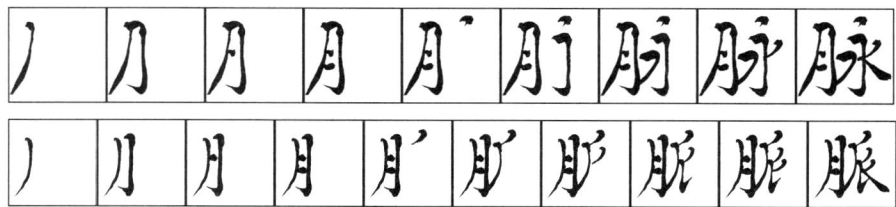

丿 刀 月 月 刖 朋 朋 脈 脈

60. 肉 〔肉〕 *ròu* Flesh

Equivalents
flesh

Significs and Stroke Counts
simplified 肉 6; complex 肉 6

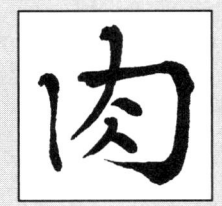

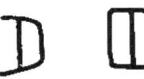

Character Composition
A pictograph portraying a lump of meat.

Explanation
The oracle-bone inscription and the lesser seal script depict a piece of rib meat; hence its original meaning is meat or flesh. Chinese characters constructed with the 肉 *ròu* component relate to the flesh, i.e., the body. When used as a component of other characters it usually takes the form of 月, which is pronounced *ròu* (or *rù* in complex characters), and should not be confused with the signific meaning "moon," which has the same form but is a different word entirely. This meaning of flesh also applies to plants and vegetables.

This graph is a signific that appears in characters denoting things related to meat or flesh. Accordingly, it occurs in many words for body organs and body parts, e.g., 脾 *pí*, spleen; 胃 *wèi*, stomach; 肝 *gān*, liver; 胆 *dǎn*, gallbladder; 脉 *mài*, vessel. Note that in certain complex character dictionaries, these characters are listed under the 6-stroke signific 肉 and are not to be found under the 4-stroke signific 月.

Combinations
脾主肉	〔脾主肉〕	*pí zhǔ ròu*	the spleen governs the flesh
筋肉	〔筋肉〕	*jīn ròu*	sinew and flesh

Stroke Sequence

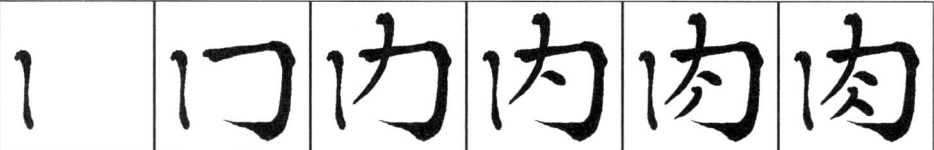

丿 冂 内 内 肉 肉 肉 肉 肉
丿 冂 内 内 肉 肉 肉 肉 肉
丿 冂 内 内 肉 肉 肉 肉 肉

61. 肌 〔肌〕 *jī* Flesh

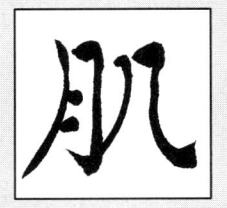

Equivalents

flesh, fleshy

Significs and Stroke Counts

simplified 月 4 + 2; complex 肉（月）6 (4) + 2

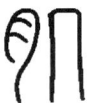

Character Composition

Signific-phonetic compound. On the left is the signific component 月 *ròu*, the flesh. On the right is the phonetic component 几 *jī*, which means a low table or stool.

Explanation

In this character the phonetic component simply contributes to the sound of the character and does not color the meaning.

Combinations

脾主肌肉	〔脾主肌肉〕	*pí zhǔ jī ròu*	the spleen governs the flesh
肌表	〔肌表〕	*jī biǎo*	fleshy exterior
生肌	〔生肌〕	*shēng jī*	engender flesh
清肌表	〔清肌表〕	*qīng jī biǎo*	clear the fleshy exterior
肌肉	〔肌肉〕	*jī ròu*	flesh; muscle

Stroke Sequence

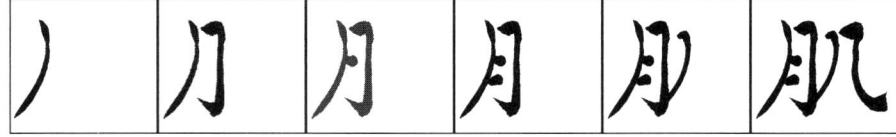

) 刀 月 月 刖 肌 肌 肌 肌 肌

62. 皮 〔皮〕 *pí* Skin

Equivalents
skin, cutaneous, hide, bark

Significs and Stroke Counts
simplified 皮 5; complex 皮 5

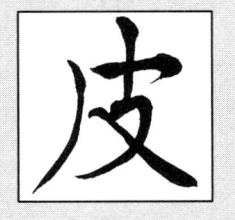

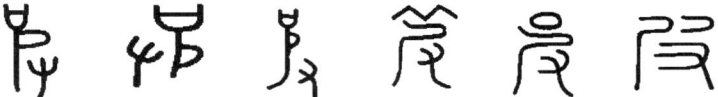

Character Composition
Pictograph portraying 又, a hand, flaying off pieces of hide.

Explanation
The ancient script of the character depicts a hand clutching the fur of an animal. Hence, its original meaning is animal fur or skin. More generally, it can be used to mean the surface of anything. Thus, it can mean skin, peel, bark, husk, hide or can connote shallowness or superficiality.

Combinations

皮色	〔皮色〕	*pí sè*	skin color
地骨皮	〔地骨皮〕	*dì gǔ pí*	lycium root bark, Lycii Cortex
七皮饮	〔七皮飲〕	*qī pí yǐn*	Seven-Peel Beverage
肺生皮毛	〔肺生皮毛〕	*fèi shēng pí máo*	lung engenders skin and [body] hair
青皮	〔青皮〕	*qīng pí*	unripe tangerine peel; Citri Reticulatae Pericarpium Viride

Stroke Sequence

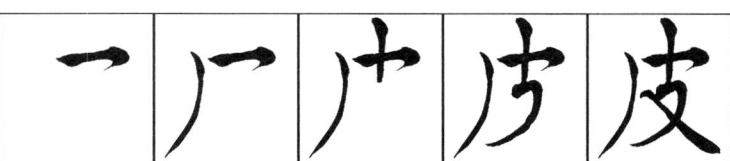

一 丆 𠂇 𠂭 皮 皮 皮 皮 皮

63. 毛〔毛〕 *máo* Body Hair

Equivalents
[body] hair, lash, down

Significs and Stroke Counts
simplified 毛 4; complex 毛 4

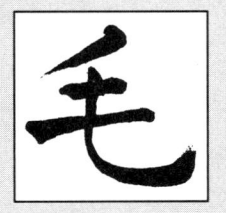

Character Composition

Pictograph portraying an animal's pelt. In the bronze inscriptions, the character 毛 *máo* depicts the shape of the hair or fur, and its original meaning is body hair (as distinct from head hair).

Explanation

In general, it indicates anything possessing the shape of hair or fur. Its meaning extends to things that are coarse, unprocessed, or unrefined. Chinese characters constructed with the 毛 *máo* component are related to hair or fur.

This character refers generally to any hair on the body, in contradistinction to 发〔髮〕 *fà* (or *fǎ*), which denotes specifically the hair of the head. The combination 皮毛 *pí máo*, skin and [body] hair, is common in Chinese; in Chinese medicine, skin and [body] hair are considered as one entity that is related to the lung.

Combinations

皮毛	〔皮毛〕	*pí máo*	skin and [body] hair
毛焦	〔毛焦〕	*máo jiāo*	parched body hair
肺主皮毛	〔肺主皮毛〕	*fèi zhǔ pí máo*	the lung governs the skin and [body] hair

Stroke Sequence

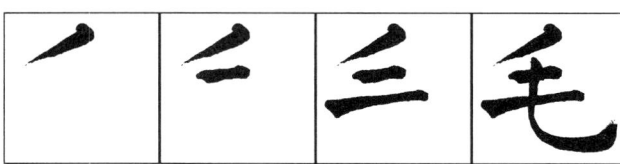

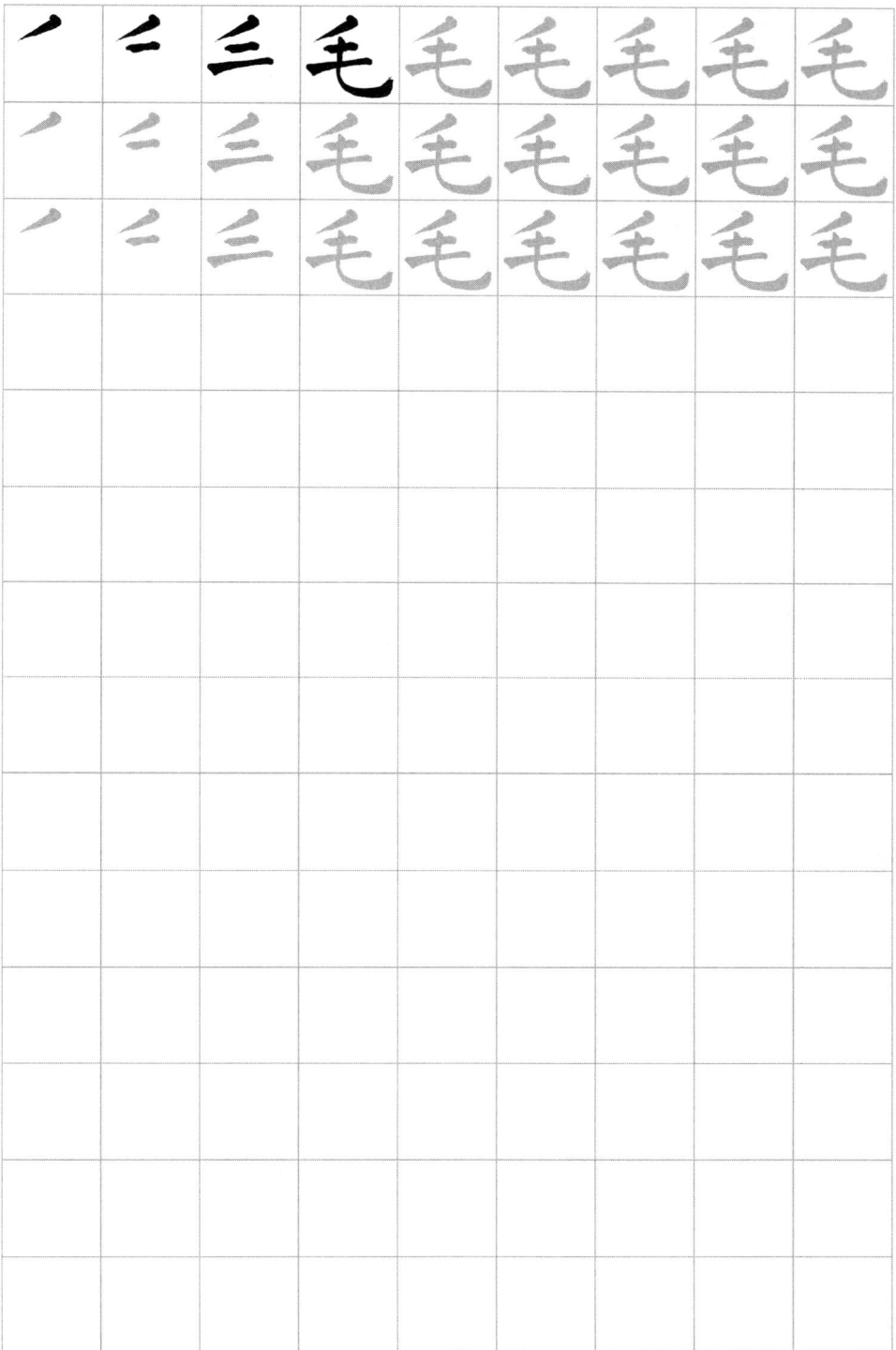

64. 骨 〔骨〕 *gǔ* Bone

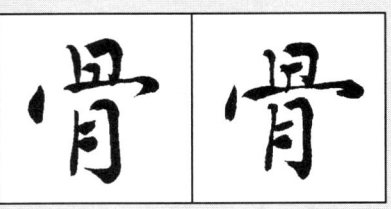

Equivalents
bone

Significs and Stroke Counts
simplified 骨 9; complex 骨 10

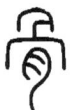

Character Composition

Pictograph. The upper part 凸 *guǎ* is supposed to represent the end of a bone shaft with a ball-like tip (e.g., the head of the femur). The lower part, 月 *roù*, flesh, was added later on to associate the character to the body.

Explanation

The ancient form of the character depicted a pile of bones, but over time the ideograph came to represent the end of a single bone. In lesser seal script, the addition of the 月 *roù* component transformed the nature of the character into an associative compound. The meaning of the character is bone.

Combinations

肾主骨	〔腎主骨〕	*shèn zhǔ gǔ*	the kidney governs the bone
筋骨	〔筋骨〕	*jīn gǔ*	sinew and bones
地骨皮	〔地骨皮〕	*dì gǔ pí*	lycium root bark; Lycii Radicis Cortex

Stroke Sequence

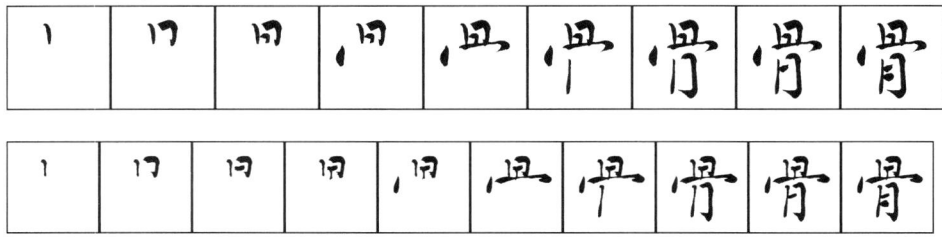

丶	冂	冋	冎	咼	骨	骨	骨	骨
丶	冂	冋	冎	咼	骨	骨	骨	骨
丶	冂	冋	冎	咼	骨	骨	骨	骨

65. 窍 [竅] *qiào* Orifice

Equivalents
 orifice

Significs and Stroke Counts
 simplified 穴 5 + 5; complex 穴 5 + 13

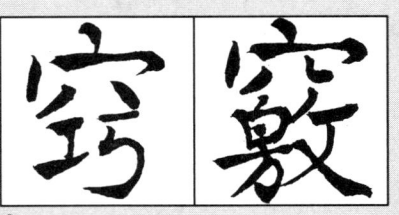

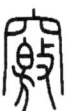

Character Composition

Signific-phonetic compound. On top is the signific component 穴 *xué*, cave or hole. Below, in the complex character, is the phonetic component 敫 *jiǎo*, which in the simplified character has been replaced with 巧 *qiǎo*, which means deft.

Explanation

Perhaps the phonetic 敫 *jiǎo* contributes to the meaning of the character. It is composed of the components sunlight, 白 *bái*, and emitting, 放 *fàng*, i.e., to shine through. Thus the whole character can be understood to mean a hole that allows light to shine through.

Combinations

上窍	[上竅]	*shàng qiào*	upper orifices
下窍	[下竅]	*xià qiào*	lower orifices
九窍	[九竅]	*jiǔ qiào*	nine orifices
七窍	[七竅]	*qī qiào*	seven orifices
心窍	[心竅]	*xīn qiào*	orifice of the heart
肾窍	[腎竅]	*shèn qiào*	orifices of the kidney
肺窍	[肺竅]	*fèi qiào*	orifice of the lung
鼻窍	[鼻竅]	*bí qiào*	nasal orifices

Stroke Sequence

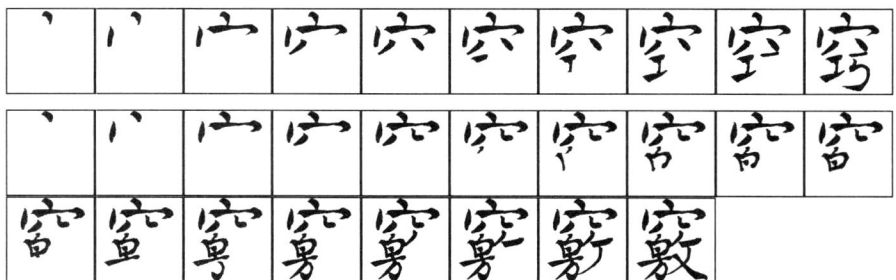

丶	宀	宀	广	宂	宍	宊	空	空	窍
丶	宀	宀	广	宂	宍	宊	空	空	窍
丶	宀	宀	广	宂	宍	宊	空	空	窍

66. 开〔開〕 *kāi* Open

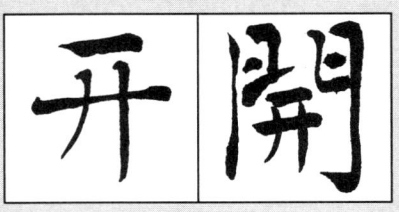

Equivalents
open

Significs and Stroke Counts
simplified 一 1 + 3; complex 門 7 + 4

Character Composition
Associative compound. The complex character is composed of the signific 門 *mén,* door, gate, and 廾 *gǒng* below means both hands reaching to and raising the door bar 一 *yī.*

Explanation
One component of the complex character is 閂 *shuān*, which is 門 *mén,* door, plus 一 *yī,* here a bar, not the numeral one. The other component is 廾 *gǒng*, which depicts a pair of hands. The hands are placed on the door bolt, indicating the action of opening. Hence, its original meaning is "to open the door." From this sense, the extended meanings include opening in general, develop, splitting, foundation, begin, arouse, and inspire. Note that the simplified character is just the hands and the door bolt.

开 *kāi* means to open, in which sense it is used in the combination 开窍 *kāi qiào*. In some contexts, it conveys the notion of freeing, e.g., 开郁 *kāi yù,* to "open depression," meaning allowing depression to dissipate.

Combinations

开水	〔開水〕	*kāi shuǐ*	boiled water
开胃	〔開胃〕	*kāi wèi*	open the stomach; increase the appetite
开窍	〔開竅〕	*kāi qiào*	open the orifices (method of treatment); open (physiology)

Stroke Sequence

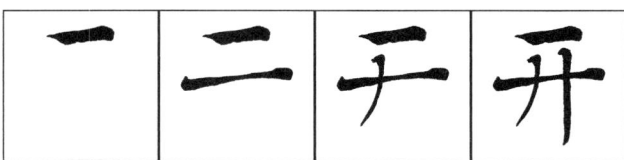

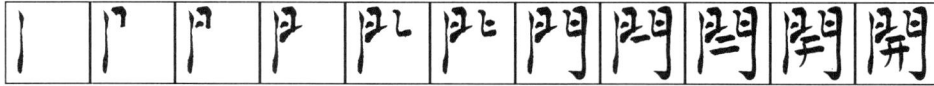

一 二 于 开 开 开 开 开 开
一 二 于 开 开 开 开 开 开
一 二 于 开 开 开 开 开 开

67. 于〔于〕 *yú* At

Equivalents
at

Significs and Stroke Counts
simplified 一 1 + 2; complex 一 1 + 2

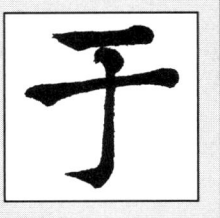

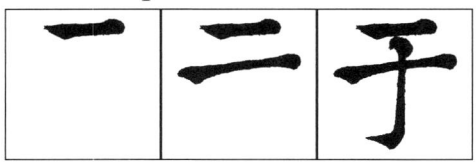

Character Composition
Loan character.

Explanation
This character originally depicted a musical instrument, the almost vertical line of the character figuratively signifying to blow through a single mouthpiece. In *Shuō Wén Jiě Zì*, this character was explained as the way the breath is exhaled evenly.

Before the modern era, another character, 於 *yú*, was a synonym of 于 *yú*, and was in fact more commonly used. When Chinese characters underwent simplification in mainland China after World War II, 于 replaced 於. Hence, in complex-character texts, one usually finds 於 and in modern simplified texts one always finds 于. Thus, 于 is often thought of as the simplified form of the character 於.

Combinations
肝开窍于目 〔肝開竅于(於)目〕 *gān kāi qiào yú mù* liver opens at the eyes
心开窍于舌 〔心開竅于(於)舌〕 *xīn kāi qiào yú shé* heart opens at the tongue
肺开窍于鼻 〔肺開竅于(於)鼻〕 *fèi kāi qiào yú bí* lung opens at the nose
肾开窍于耳 〔腎開竅于(於)耳〕 *shèn kāi qiào yú ér* kidney opens at the ears

Stroke Sequence

| 一 | 二 | 于 |

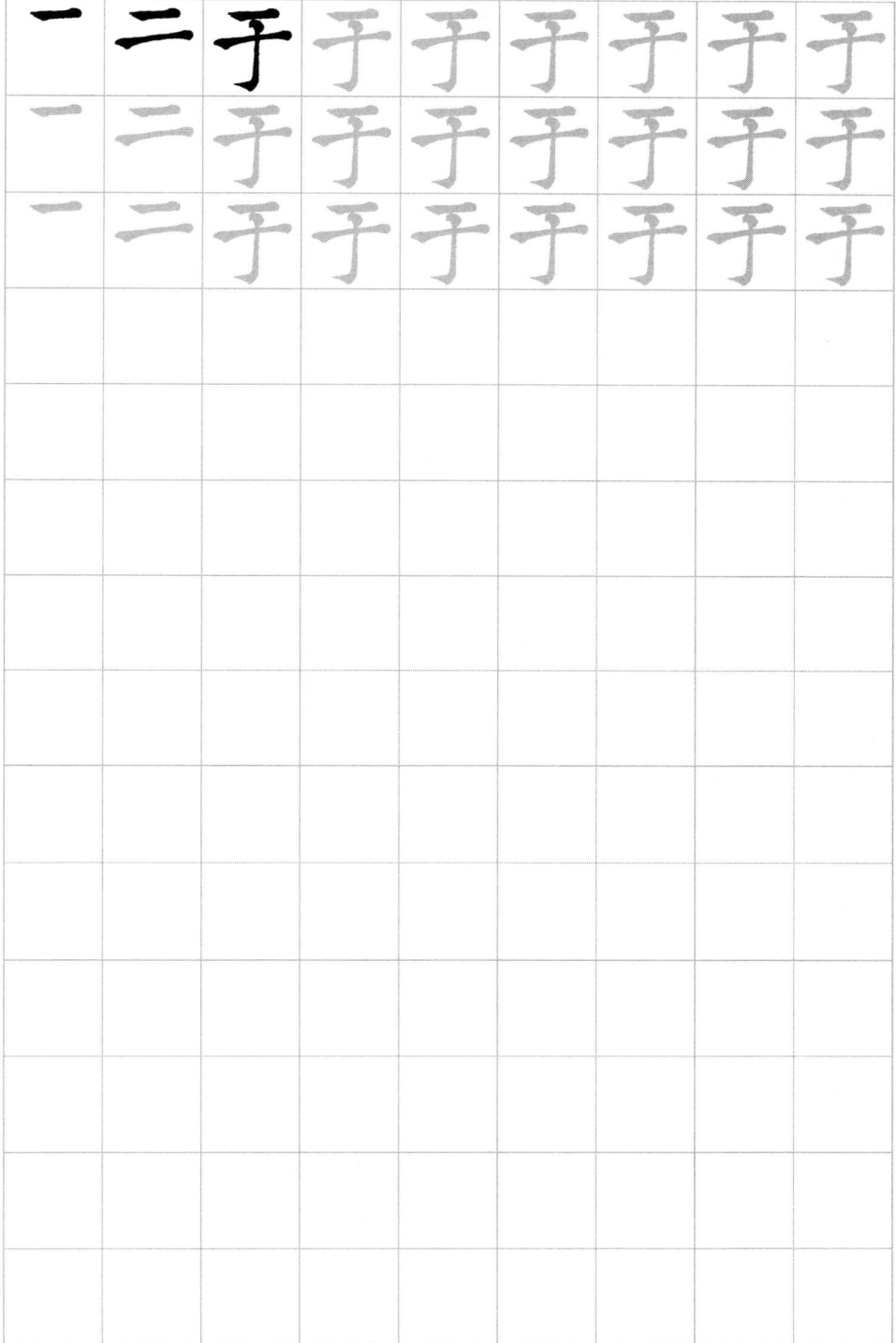

68. 目〔目〕 *mù* Eye

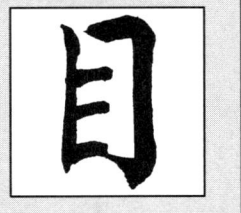

Equivalents
eye, vision

Significs and Stroke Counts
simplified 目 5; complex 目 5

Character Composition

A pictographic representation of the eye, with the two middle bars delineating the iris.

Explanation

The oracle-bone form of this character depicts an eye, and its original meaning is the eye. It is also used as a verb: to look, looking, watching. The meanings of 目 *mù* also extend to mean the mesh of a fishing net as well as an array of other extended meanings such as entry, clause, and sub clauses. Most Chinese characters constructed with the component 目 *mù* are related to the eye, or the function of the eye, such as sight and vision.

目 *mù* means the physical eye. 明目 *míng mù* means "brighten the eyes," implying an improvement in vision.

Combinations

肝主目	〔肝主目〕	*gān zhǔ mù*	liver governs the eyes
目黄	〔目黃〕	*mù huáng*	yellowing of the eyes
风热目赤	〔風熱目赤〕	*fēng rè mù chì*	wind-heat red eye
肝开窍于目	〔肝開竅于(於)目〕	*gān kāi qiào yú mù*	the liver opens at the eyes

Stroke Sequence

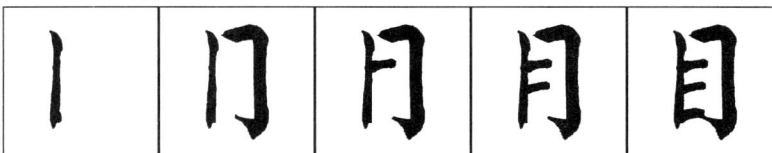

丨 冂 冃 月 目 目 目 目 目
丨 冂 冃 目 目 目 目 目 目
丨 冂 冃 目 目 目 目 目 目

69. 舌〔舌〕 *shé* Tongue

Equivalents

tongue

Significs and Stroke Counts

simplified 舌 6; complex 舌 6

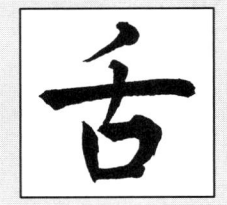

Character Composition

A pictograph representing the tongue sticking out of the mouth.

Explanation

In the oracle-bone inscriptions, the character 舌 *shé* is a depiction of a tongue. The meaning of the character extends to many aspects of speech. Any Chinese character constructed with the component of 舌 *shé* is related to the functions of the tongue: taste and speech.

Combinations

木舌	〔木舌〕	*mù shé*	wooden tongue
青舌	〔青舌〕	*qīng shé*	green-blue tongue
木风舌	〔木風舌〕	*mù fēng shé*	wood wind tongue
血瘀舌下	〔血瘀舌下〕	*xuè yū shé xià*	blood stasis under the tongue
心开窍于舌	〔心開竅于(於)舌〕	*xīn kāi qiào yú shé*	the heart opens into the tongue

Stroke Sequence

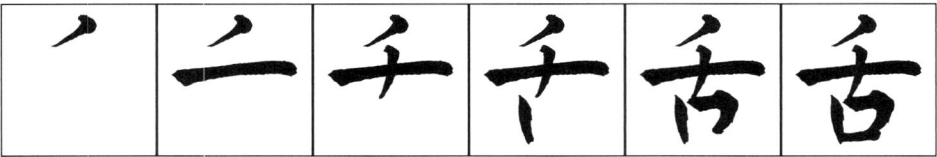

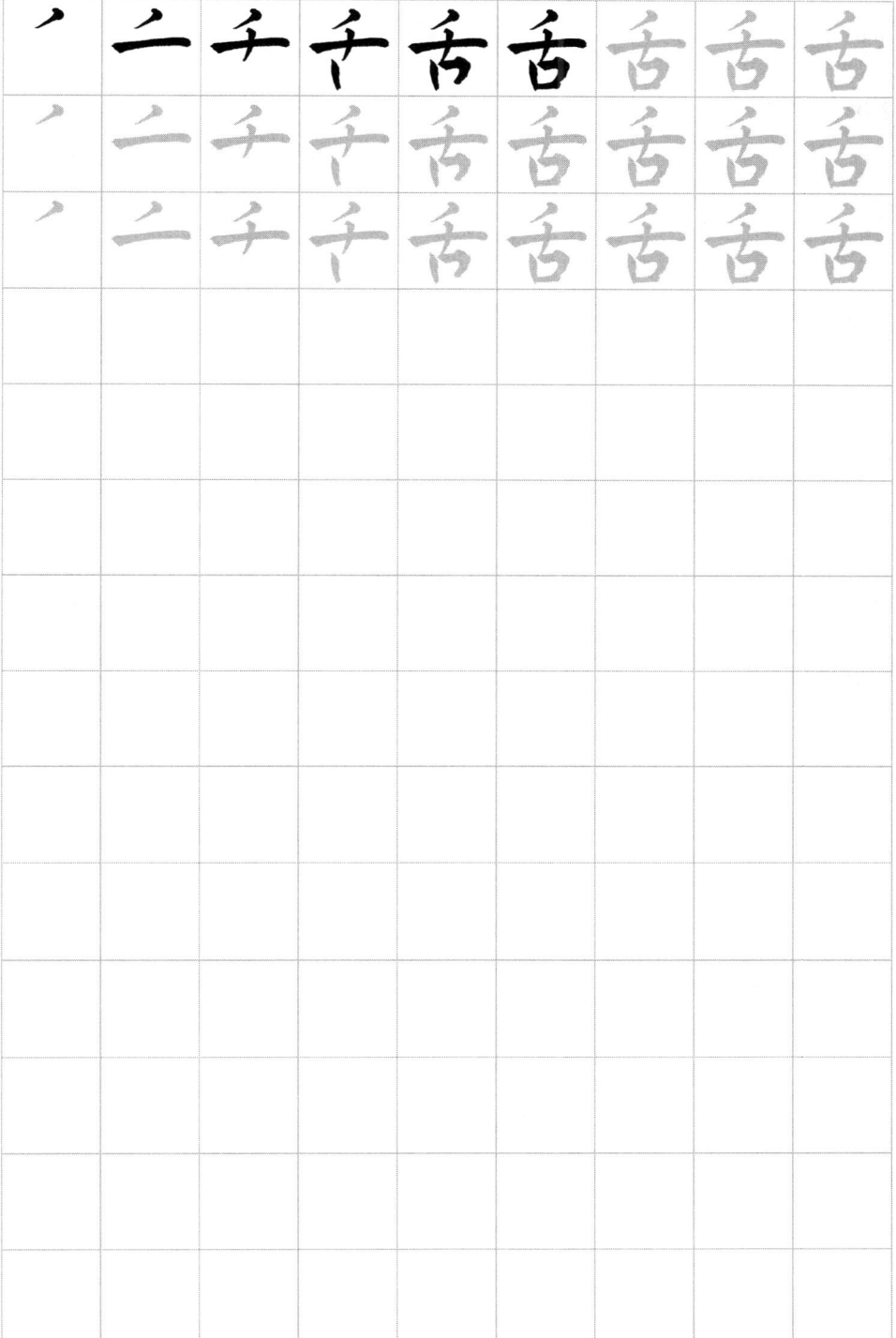

70. 口 〔口〕 *kǒu* Mouth

Equivalents

mouth, opening

Significs and Stroke Counts

simplified 口 3; complex 口 3

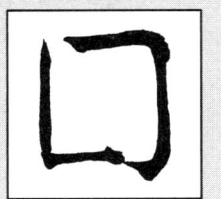

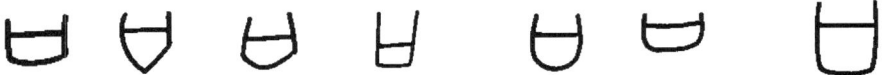

Character Composition

A pictograph depicting the mouth.

Explanation

口 *kǒu* means mouth, and by extension an opening. In Chinese medicine it is used in both these senses. Chinese characters constructed with the component 口 *kǒu* tend to be related to the mouth, eating, or speech. In modern Chinese, mouth is usually referred to as 嘴 *zuǐ* or 嘴巴 *zuǐ bā*.

Combinations

脉口	〔脈口〕	*mài kǒu*	vessel opening
口水	〔口水〕	*kǒu shuǐ*	saliva
口气	〔口氣〕	*kǒu qì*	smell of the breath
口鼻气热	〔口鼻氣熱〕	*kǒu bí qì rè*	hot breath from the nose and mouth
脾开窍于口	〔脾開竅于(於)口〕	*pí kāi qiào yú kǒu*	the spleen opens into the mouth

Stroke Sequence

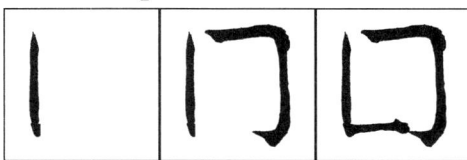

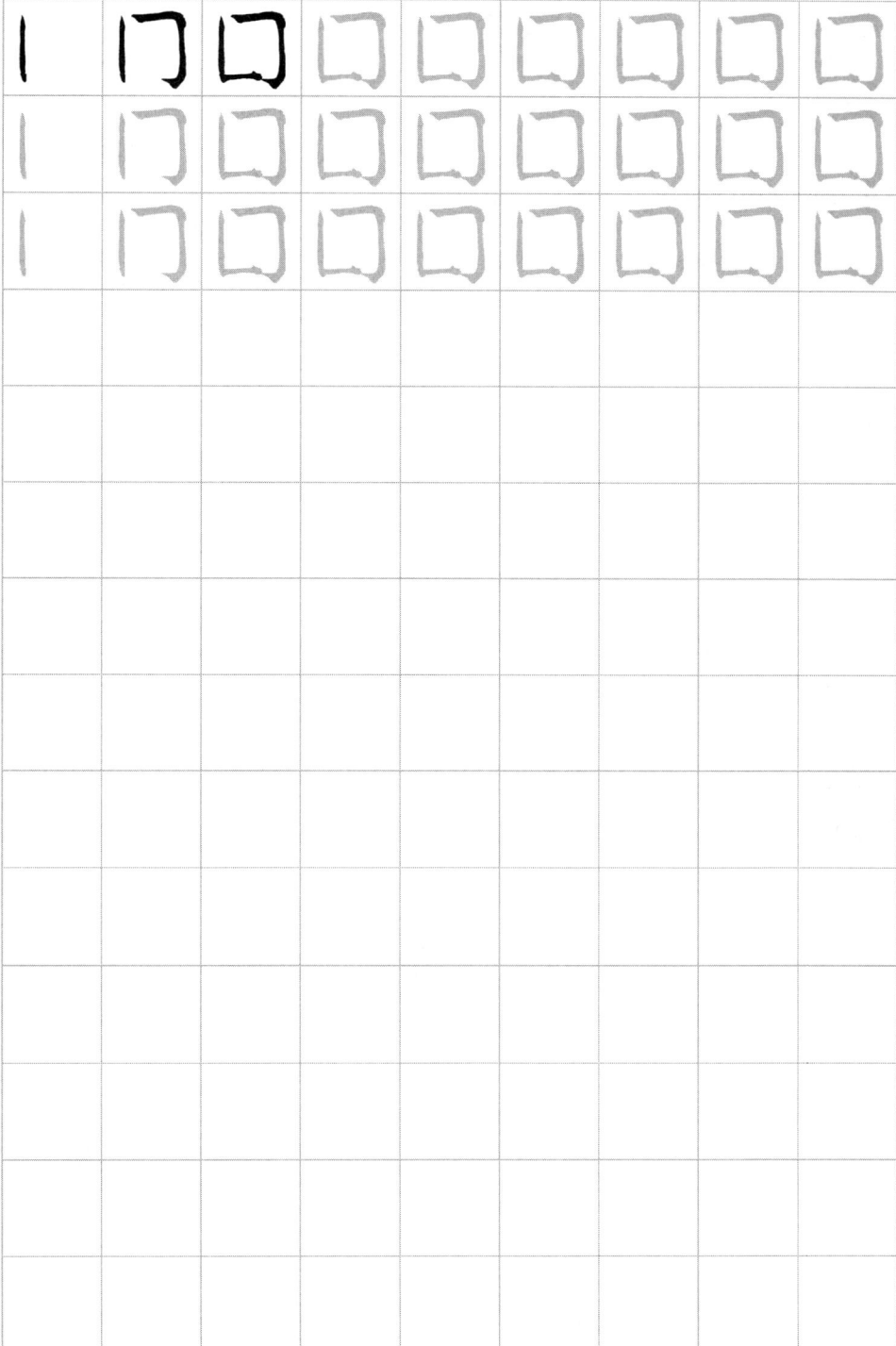

71. 鼻〔鼻〕 *bí* Nose

Equivalents
nose, nasal

Significs and Stroke Counts
simplified 鼻 14; complex 鼻 14

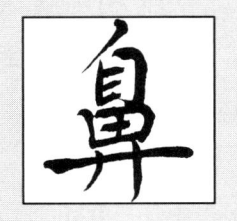

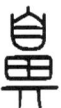

Character Composition

Signific-phonetic compound composed of the signific component 自 *zì* on top and the phonetic 畀 *bì* below.

Explanation

The oracle-bone form of the character 自 *zì* was a pictograph of a nose, and it was the original character for nose. However, the character 自 *zì* was widely used for its extended meaning, the self. Therefore, the character 鼻 *bí* was invented to isolate the original meaning from the extended meaning; hence, 鼻 *bí*, the nose.

In Chinese medicine, the nose is usually referred to as 鼻 *bí*. In the modern spoken language, it is usually referred to as 鼻子 *bí zi*.

Combinations

鼻赤	〔鼻赤〕	*bí chì*	red nose (drinker's nose)
鼻窍	〔鼻竅〕	*bí qiào*	nose orifices
肺主鼻	〔肺主鼻〕	*fèi zhǔ bí*	lung governs the nose
肺开窍于鼻	〔肺開竅于(於)鼻〕	*fèi kāi qiào yú bí*	the lung opens at the nose
口鼻气热	〔口鼻氣熱〕	*kǒu bí qì rè*	hot breath from the nose and mouth

Stroke Sequence

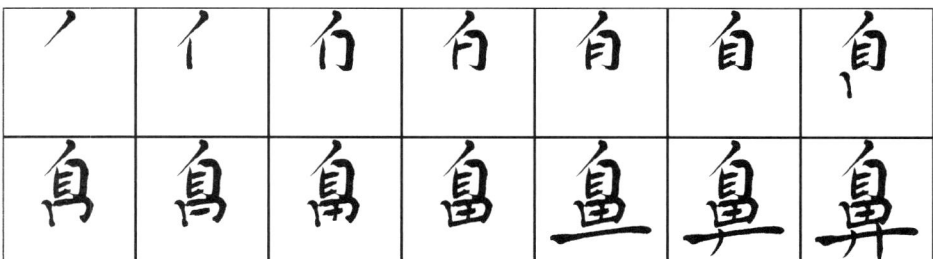

72. 耳〔耳〕 ěr Ear

Equivalents

ear

Significs and Stroke Counts

simplified 耳 6; complex 耳 6

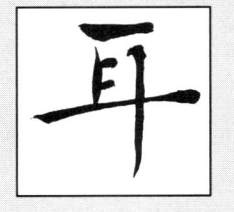

Character Composition

Pictograph. The oracle-bone form of the character depicts an ear, and its original meaning is the ear.

Explanation

Chinese characters constructed with the component of 耳 ěr are typically related to the ear, or the sense or function of hearing.

In Chinese medicine, the ear is usually referred to as 耳 ěr. In the modern spoken language, it is usually referred to as 耳朵 ěr duo, 朵 usually otherwise being a measure word for flowers, in which case it is pronounced duǒ.

Combinations

风耳	〔風耳〕	fēng ěr	wind ear
白木耳	〔白木耳〕	bái mù ěr	tremella; Tremella
血瘀耳窍	〔血瘀耳竅〕	xuè yū ěr qiào	blood stasis in the ear orifice
肾开窍于耳	〔腎開竅于(於)耳〕	shèn kāi qiào yú ěr	the kidney opens at the ears

Stroke Sequence

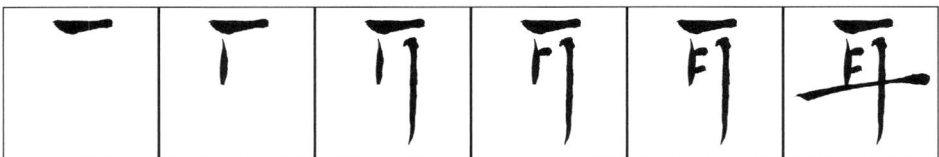

一 丆 厅 斤 斤 耳 耳 耳 耳
一 丆 厅 斤 斤 耳 耳 耳 耳
一 丆 厅 斤 斤 耳 耳 耳 耳

73. 经〔經〕 *jīng* Channel

Equivalents
channel, river, canon, menses

Significs and Stroke Counts
simplified 纟 3 + 5; complex 糸（糸）6 + 7

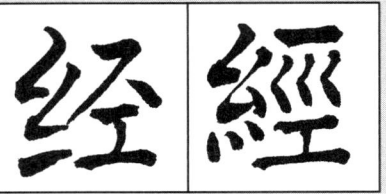

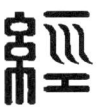

Character Composition
Associative compound. The signific on the left is silk 糸 *sī*. On the right, the phonetic 巠 *jīng* also serves as a signific. As well as meaning the warp of a fabric, 巠 *jīng* is the character used by geomancers to denote the flow of water underground. In other characters with 巠 *jīng* as the phonetic it has the meaning of straight.

Explanation
This character is frequently used in Chinese medical texts and has many meanings, including channel, river (as a body of water and also the river points in acupuncture), canon, and menses. While most reference works explain this character depicts silk on the left with a loom on the right and originally meant the warp of a fabric, the combination of significs can be understood to speak volumes about the nature of channels. That is, the channels can be thought of as carrying qì and blood through the body like groundwater passes under the earth. Moreover, the silk signific reminds us that if we dissect a body and look for the channels, they are not to be found; that is, they have the subtle nature of a single strand of silk.

Combinations
内经	〔内經〕	*nèi jīng*	Inner Canon
大肠经	〔大腸經〕	*dà cháng jīng*	large intestine channel; LI
六经	〔六經〕	*liù jīng*	six channels

Stroke Sequence

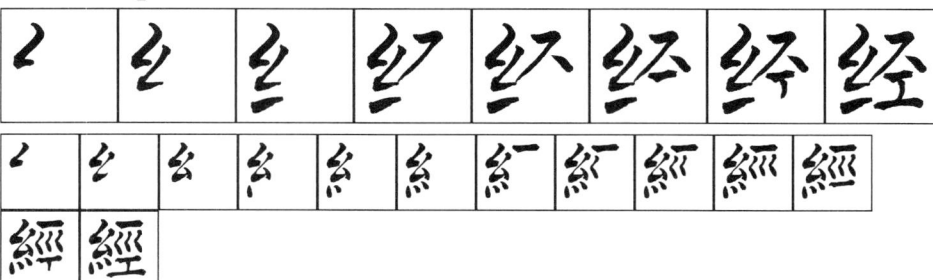

74. 络 〔絡〕 *luò* Network, Net

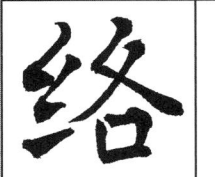 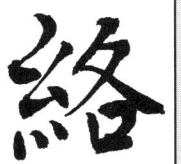

Equivalents
network, net

Significs and Stroke Counts
simplified 纟 3 + 6 complex 糸（糹）6 + 6

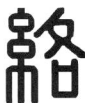

Character Composition
Signific-phonetic complex.

Explanation
This character takes its meaning from the silk signific on the left and its pronunciation from 各 *gē* on the right. It originally meant unreeled silk, hemp, or cotton fiber, and from its associations with stringy fibers came to be used in Chinese medicine as a noun that means network and as a verb that means to net.

Combinations

经络	〔經絡〕	*jīng luò*	channels and network vessels
大络	〔大絡〕	*dà luò*	great network vessel
心经络于小肠	〔心經絡于小腸〕	*xīn jīng luò yú xiǎo cháng*	the heart channel nets the small intestine
舌下络脉	〔舌下絡脈〕	*shé xià luò mài*	sublingual network vessels
清络饮	〔清絡飲〕	*qīng luò yǐn*	Network-Clearing Beverage

Stroke Sequence

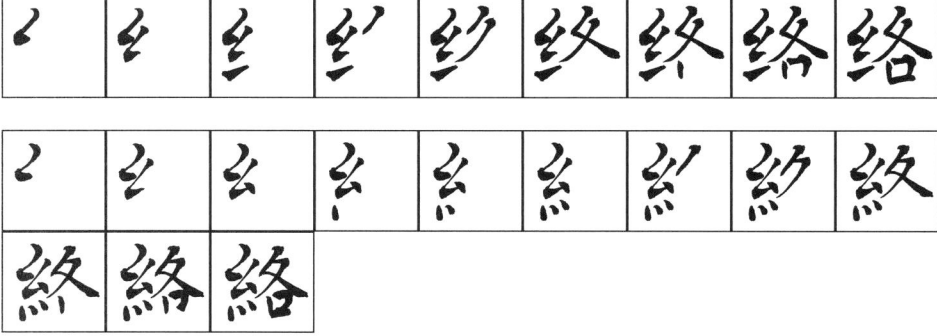

丶 纟 纟 纟 纱 纹 终 络 络

75. 面〔面〕 *miàn* Face

Equivalents

face, facial

Significs and Stroke Counts

simplified 面 9; complex 面 9

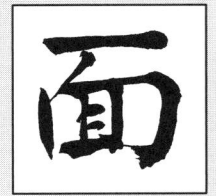

Character Composition

Pictograph. The oracle-bone form of this character depicts an eye in the center of the outlines of a face. Thus its original meaning is the face.

Explanation

Since the depiction of 面 *miàn* indicates the whole front of the head, the meaning of the character extends to include frontal, external, exterior.

面 *miàn* is the word usually used in Chinese medical terminology to represent the idea of face. In the modern spoken language, it is 脸 *liǎn*.

Combinations

面色	〔面色〕	*miàn sè*	facial complexion
面色黄	〔面色黃〕	*miàn sè huáng*	yellow facial complexion
面赤	〔面赤〕	*miàn chì*	red face
赤面风	〔赤面風〕	*chì miàn fēng*	red face wind

Stroke Sequence

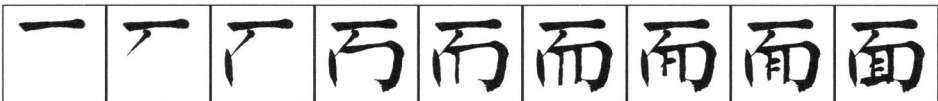

一 丆 厂 丂 而 而 而 而 面

76. 色〔色〕 *sè* Color

Equivalents
color, complexion

Significs and Stroke Counts
simplified 色 6; complex 色 6

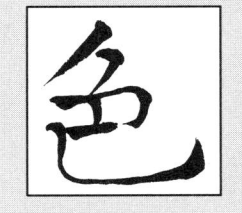

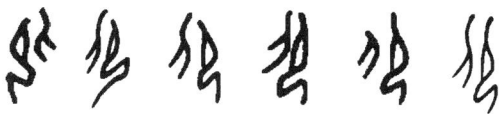

Character Composition

Associative compound. On top is the variant form of the character 人 *rén*, man. On the bottom is 卪 *jié*, a seal. However, certain sources use 刀 *dāo*, a knife, as the signific of the simplified character.

Explanation

The color of the face corresponds with the feeling of the heart, as the stamp reproduces the seal. By extension and in compounds with other words this character often refers to emotions that result in changes in the color of the face (the flush arising from passion or sexual pleasure) or to color in general.

In modern spoken Chinese, color as an independent concept is usually 颜色 *yán sè*.

Combinations

面色	〔面色〕	*miàn sè*	facial complexion
面色白	〔面色白〕	*miàn sè bái*	white facial complexion
面色黄	〔麵色黃〕	*miàn sè huáng*	yellow facial complexion
面色黑	〔面色黑〕	*miàn sè hēi*	black facial complexion

Stroke Sequence

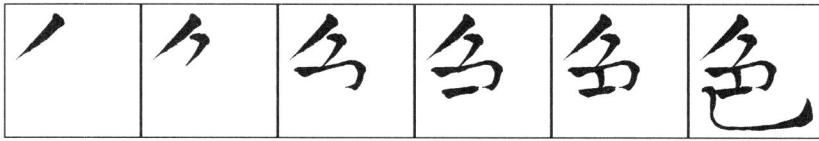

丿 ⼓ 厶 刍 刍 色 色 色 色

77. 青〔青〕 *qīng* Green-Blue

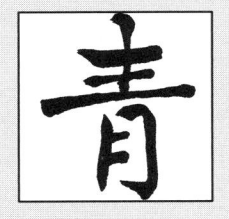

Equivalents

green-blue, black

Significs and Stroke Counts

simplified 青 8; complex 青 8

  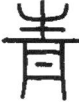

Character Composition

Associative compound. The character is composed of 生 *shēng*, life and growth, on top, and 丹 *dān* on the bottom.

Explanation

The oracle-bone form of 丹 *dān* is the depiction of a tool used for grinding and mixing colors. The character came to mean the color of one frequently used ingredient, both in painting and alchemy, cinnabar. Thus, in time the extended meaning of 丹 *dān* included the elixir of longevity, which often involved cinnabar ground with such a tool. The combination of these two components gives rise to the meaning of youth, which suggests that life is rooted in 丹 *dān*, the elixir.

The change from 丹 *dān* to 月 *yuè* was only in the form, not in meaning.

青 *qīng* is the color of growing plants (note that our word "green" is related to "grow" for the same reason). It also came to denote blue as well as black. In modern Chinese, the standard word for green is 绿 *lǜ*.

Combinations

面色青	〔面色青〕	*miàn sè qīng*	green-blue facial complexion
舌青	〔舌青〕	*shé qīng*	green-blue tongue
大青	〔大青〕	*dà qīng*	isatis, Isatidis Folium; lit., "big green"
青筋	〔青筋〕	*qīng jīn*	veins (showing on the surface of the body)

Stroke Sequence

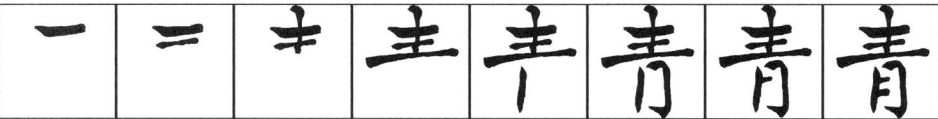

一	二	三	丯	丰	青	青	青	青	青
一	二	三	丯	丰	青	青	青	青	青
一	二	三	丯	丰	青	青	青	青	青

78. 赤 〔赤〕 *chì* Red

Equivalents
red

Significs and Stroke Counts
simplified 赤 7; complex 赤 7

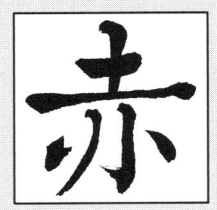

      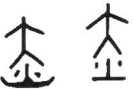 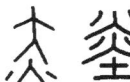

Character Composition

Associative compound. The original character was 大 *dà*, representing a human being, with fire 火 *huǒ* below it.

Explanation

The notion of red derives from the fact that fire causes the skin to turn red. The ancient form of the character depicts a person standing on top of fire; hence its original meaning is fire. Since the flame of the fire is red, the character 赤 *chì* came to mean the color red. 赤 *chì* also means nakedness.

In the modern language, 赤 *chì* has now been replaced by 红 *hóng*. In Chinese medicine, 赤 *chì* continues to be the standard, although 红 *hóng* is also found.

Combinations

目赤	〔目赤〕	*mù chì*	red eyes
面赤	〔面赤〕	*miàn chì*	red face
面色赤	〔面色赤〕	*miàn sè chì*	red facial complexion
鼻赤	〔鼻赤〕	*bí chì*	red nose
赤肉	〔赤肉〕	*chì ròu*	red flesh
赤土	〔赤土〕	*chì tǔ*	alternate Chinese name for hematite (代赭石 *dài zhě shí*)

Stroke Sequence

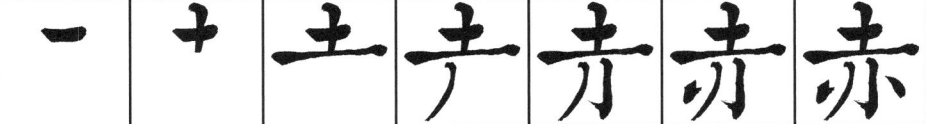

一 十 土 ナ 亦 赤 赤 赤 赤

79. 黄 〔黃〕 *huáng* Yellow

Equivalents
  yellow, jaundice

Significs and Stroke Counts
  simplified 黄 11; complex 黃 12

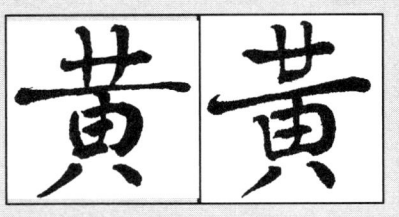

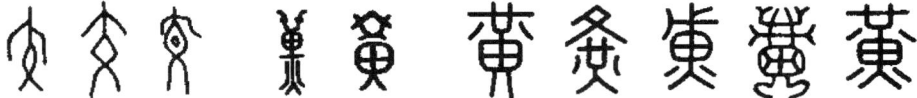

Character Composition

Associative compound/loan character. In the complex characters, this character is a single signific unto itself.

Explanation

The oracle-bone inscription depicts an ornamental jade that was worn hanging around a person's waist. Hence its original meaning is "waist jade." However, the character was borrowed to mean the color yellow, and its original meaning slowly faded away. There is another character invented to mean this specific original meaning of jade, 璜 *huáng*. An alternative reading of the etymology is based on the fact that in the old forms the character clearly indicates the middle section of the human body and thus associates the concept of the center, long symbolized in China by the color yellow. Yellow is the color of the ploughed earth, and in *Shuō Wén Jiě Zì*, it states that the character follows from the signific 田 *tián,* field and 光 *guāng*, brightness of the sun, which lends to the earth its yellow hue.

Combinations

面黄	〔面黃〕	*miàn huáng*	yellow face
面色黄	〔面色黃〕	*miàn sè huáng*	yellow facial complexion
目黄	〔目黃〕	*mù huáng*	yellowing of the eyes
大黄	〔大黃〕	*dà huáng*	rhubarb, Rhei Radix et Rhizoma
地黄	〔地黃〕	*dì huáng*	rehmannia, Rehmanniae Radix

Stroke Sequence

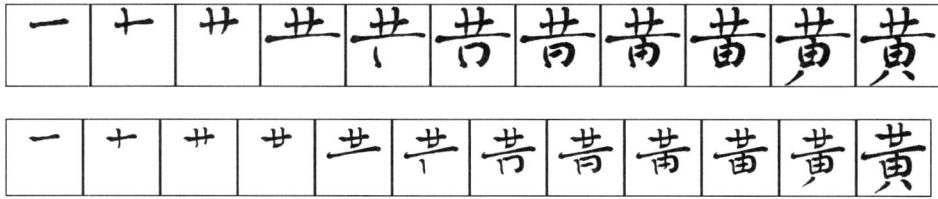

| 一 | 十 | 卄 | 丗 | 쓰 | 꿈 | 昔 | 苗 | 苗 | 黃 | 黃 |

80. 白〔白〕 *bái* White

Equivalents

white

Significs and Stroke Counts

simplified 白 5; complex 白 5

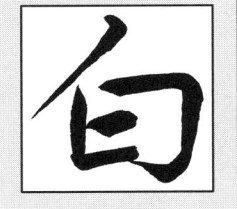

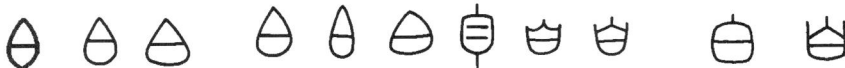

Character Composition

Ideograph. The character is composed of 日 *rì,* sun, with an extra mark to distinguish it.

Explanation

The interpretation of this character based on the lesser seal inscription suggests that the meaning develops from the appearance of the sun at dawn. This meaning is represented by a small dot on the top of the sun, i.e., the dawn, when the eastern sky becomes white. However, both oracle-bone inscription and bronze inscription of 白 *bái* depict an almost oval-shaped grain of rice. Hence, the original meaning of 白 *bái* came from the white color of rice. By extension its meaning includes pure, clear, and understanding. It also can be used as a verb that means to articulate clearly, to profess.

Combinations

面白	〔面白〕	*miàn bái*	white face
面色白	〔面色白〕	*miàn sè bái*	white facial complexion
赤白	〔赤白〕	*chì bái*	red and white

Stroke Sequence

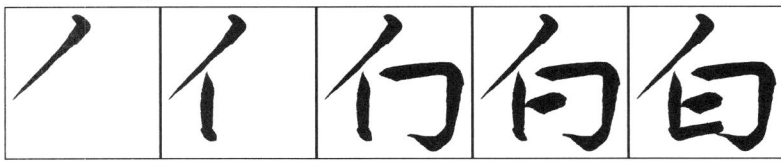

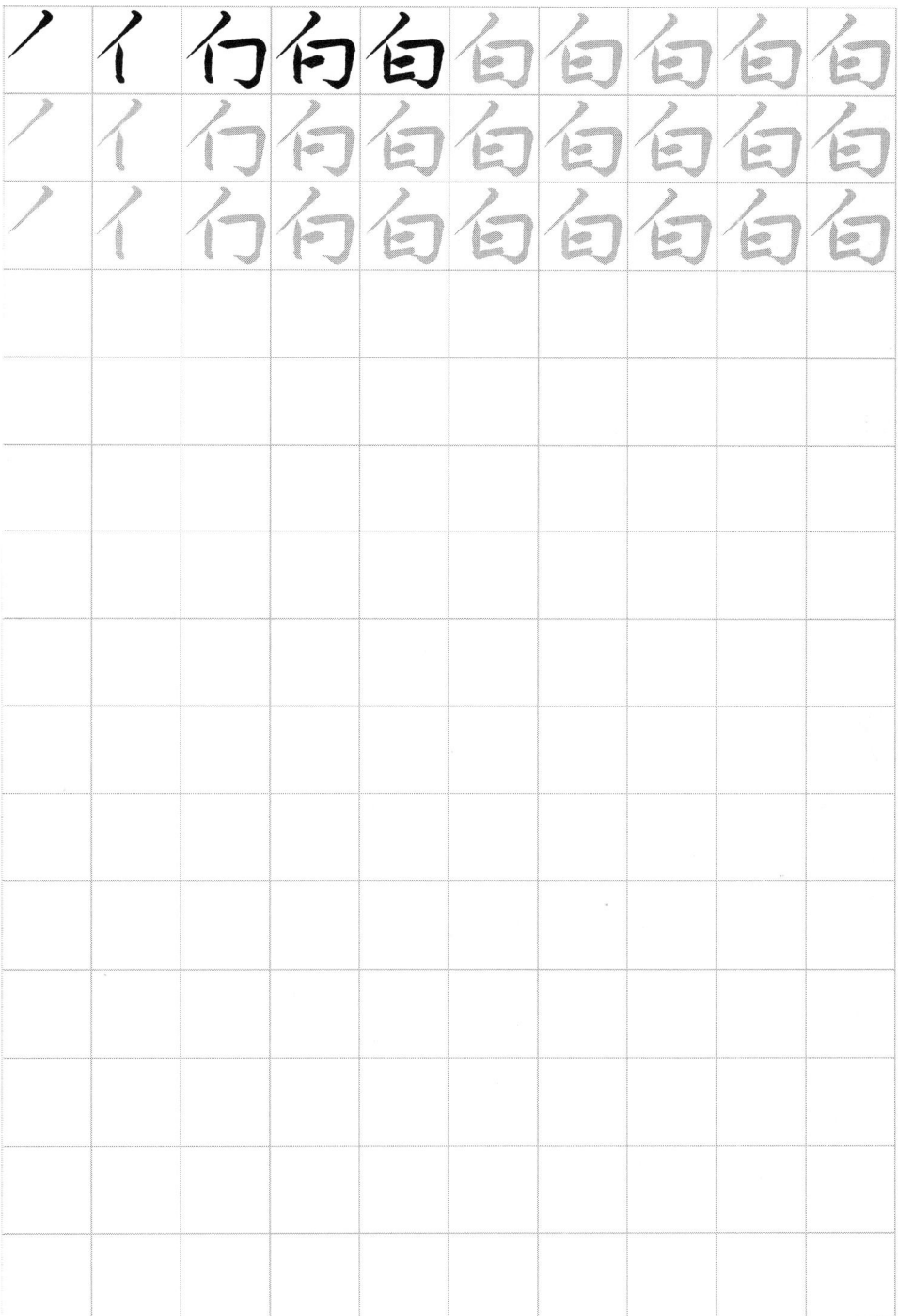

81. 黑〔黑〕 *hēi* Black

Equivalents

black

Significs and Stroke Counts

simplified 黑 12; complex 黑 12

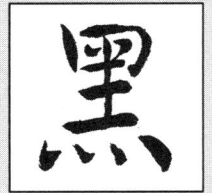

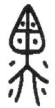 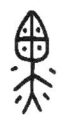 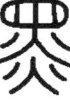

Character Composition

Pictograph of a flame rising up and venting through a chimney, i.e., the color of what has been charred by fire.

Explanation

The oracle-bone form of this character depicts a person who is being enveloped by smoke from a fire. Its original meaning is to be covered with smoke. This meaning was later extended to include the color black. By analogy, it was extended to include meanings such as the darkness of night and privacy.

Combinations

面黑	〔面黑〕	*miàn hēi*	black face
面色黑	〔面色黑〕	*miàn sè hēi*	black facial complexion
黑风	〔黑風〕	*hēi fēng*	black wind

Stroke Sequence

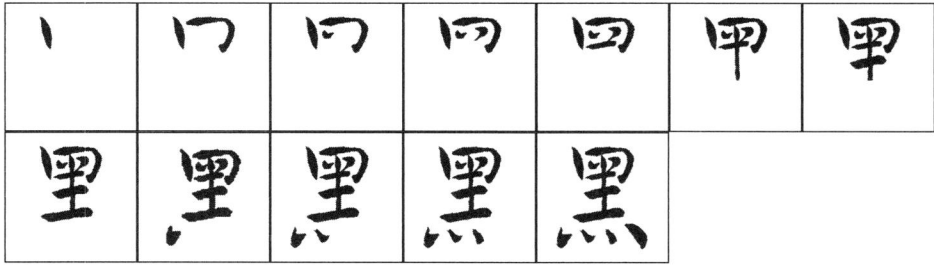

丶	冂	冂	冋	曰	甲	甲	里	里	黑	黑	黑
丶	冂	冂	冋	曰	甲	甲	里	里	黑	黑	黑
丶	冂	冂	冋	曰	甲	甲	里	里	黑	黑	黑

82. 泪〔淚〕 *lèi* Tears

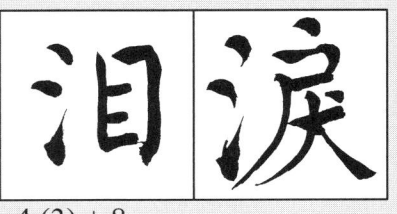

Equivalents

tears

Significs and Stroke Counts

simplified 氵 3 + 5; complex 水（氵）4 (3) + 8

Character Composition

Associative compound; however, the complex form of the character is a signific-phonetic compound.

Explanation

Originally this character was drawn like the simplified character is drawn today. On the left is the signific component 氵 *shuǐ*, water. On the right is the component 目 *mù*, the eyes. The combination of the two components gives the idea of the water of the eyes. Hence the character means tears.

However, at some point in history the complex form of the character came into use. It is simply the signific component 氵 *shuǐ*, water, with a phonetic component 戾 *lì*.

Note that the printed font used here presents a variant of the complex character that students should learn to recognize when reading. But, in handwritten Chinese, the strokes should be made as presented in the Stroke Sequence below.

Combinations

泪水	〔淚水〕	*lèi shuǐ*	tears
泪窍	〔淚竅〕	*lèi qiào*	tear orifices
泪热	〔淚熱〕	*lèi rè*	hot tears

Stroke Sequence

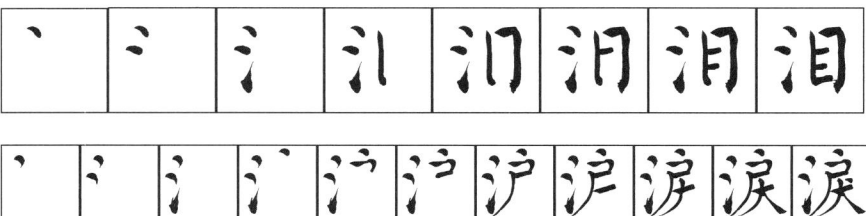

泪

83. 汗〔汗〕 *hàn* Sweat

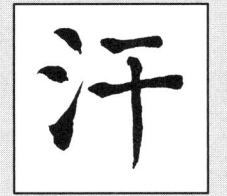

Equivalents

sweat(ing)

Significs and Stroke Counts

simplified 氵 3 + 3; complex 水（氵）4 (3) + 3

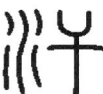

Character Composition

Signific-phonetic compound. On the left is the signific 氵 *shuǐ,* and on the right is the phonetic 干 *gān.*

Explanation

This compound represents the body fluid.

Combinations

汗气	〔汗氣〕	*hàn qì*	smell of sweat
大汗	〔大汗〕	*dà hàn*	great sweating
黄汗	〔黃汗〕	*huáng hàn*	yellow sweat

Stroke Sequence

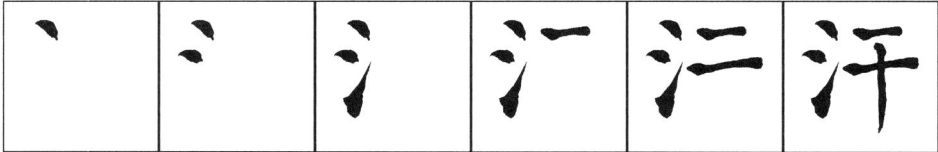

汗

84. 涎 〔涎〕 *xián* Drool

Equivalents
drool

Significs and Stroke Counts
simplified 氵 3 + 6; complex 水（氵）4 (3) + 7

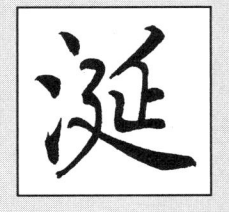

 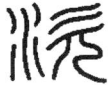

Character Composition

Signific-phonetic compound. On the left is the water signific 氵 *shuǐ*; on the right is 延 *yán*, which is a phonetic element, but which may also contribute to the meaning.

Explanation

The phonetic component on the right is 延 *yán*, a dragging motion. It is composed of 廴 *yǐn*, and 止 *zhǐ,* here meaning the foot. Thus, the meaning of 延 *yán* becomes "extension," "extend," or "prolong," which could be thought of as part of the original meaning of 涎 *xián*, "drool."

Note that while the simplified and complex characters look the same, the phonetic is drawn with 6 strokes in the simplified and 7 strokes in the complex. (The difference is clearly illustrated in the stroke sequence below.) Beginning students should not put too much effort into memorizing this sort of difference; when using dictionaries later, however, it will be important to recall that there are many fine details to determining stroke counts.

Combinations

涎唾	〔涎唾〕	*xián tuò*	drool-spittle
涎为脾液	〔涎為脾液〕	*xián wéi pí yè*	drool is the humor of the spleen
痰涎	〔痰涎〕	*tán xián*	phlegm-drool
涎下	〔涎下〕	*xián xià*	drooling

Stroke Sequence

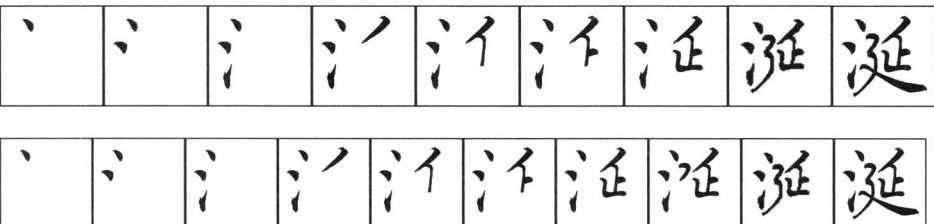

涎

85. 涕 〔涕〕 *tì* Snivel

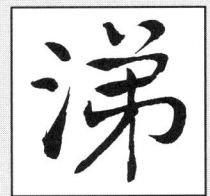

Equivalents

snivel, nasal mucus, tears

Significs and Stroke Counts

simplified 氵 3 + 7; complex 水（氵）4 (3) + 7

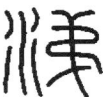

Character Composition

Signific-phonetic compound. On the left is the water signific 氵 *shuǐ*; on the right is the phonetic 弟 *dì*.

Explanation

The phonetic connotes the meaning of a sequence of action, from which derives the sense of the younger brother, i.e., the one who follows in sequence. From the combination with 氵 *shuǐ*, the water on the left side, there develops the meaning of water that follows in sequence, such as tears and snivel.

Combinations

鼻涕	〔鼻涕〕	*bí tì*	snivel; nasal mucus
鼻涕黄	〔鼻涕黃〕	*bí tì huáng*	yellow snivel; yellow nasal mucus
鼻涕黄浊	〔鼻涕黃濁〕	*bí tì huáng zhuó*	turbid yellow snivel (nasal mucus)
鼻涕清	〔鼻涕清〕	*bí tì qīng*	clear snivel (nasal mucus)

Stroke Sequence

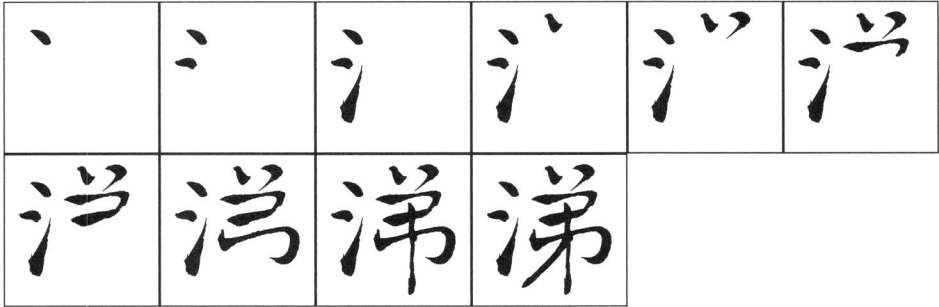

丶 丶 氵 氵 氵 泸 泸 涕 涕 涕

86. 唾 〔唾〕 *tuò* Spittle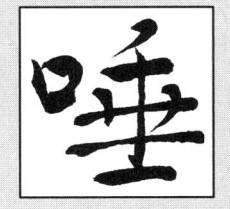

Equivalents

spittle

Significs and Stroke Counts

simplified ☐ 3 + 8; complex ☐ 3 + 8

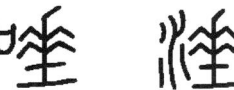

Character Composition

Signific-phonetic compound. On the left is the mouth signific ☐ *kǒu;* on the right is the phonetic 垂 *chuí*.

Explanation

The phonetic component on the right, 垂 *chuí*, depicts a plant with drooping leaves or fruit. The meaning of spittle comes from the combination of this with the mouth signific, i.e., that which falls from the mouth. In the lesser seal script, the character was composed of the mouth or water on the left side symbolizing the liquid of the mouth, i.e., the spittle. It is also used as a verb: to spit, spitting.

Combinations

涎唾	〔涎唾〕	*xián tuò*	drool and spittle
唾液	〔唾液〕	*tuò yè*	spittle humor
唾血	〔唾血〕	*tuò xuè*	spitting of blood

Stroke Sequence

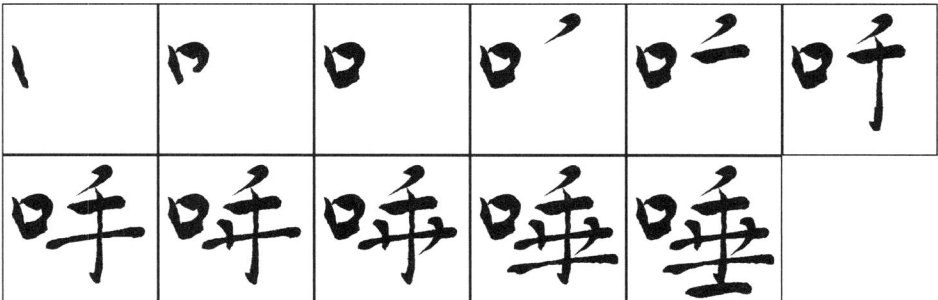

丶	口	口	口丿	口一	吁	呼	呼	唾	唾
丶	口	口	口丿	口一	吁	呼	呼	唾	唾
丶	口	口	口丿	口一	吁	呼	呼	唾	唾

87. 因 〔因〕 *yīn* Cause

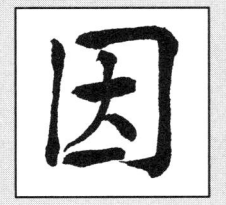

Equivalents
cause

Significs and Stroke Counts
simplified ☐ 3 + 3; complex ☐ 3 + 3

       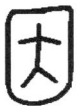

Character Composition
Pictograph/ideograph showing a man lying flat on a mat.

Explanation
The ancient form of the character depicts a man lying flat on a mat with both arms and legs spread wide. Thus, its original meaning is "mat." It is the original character for 茵 *yīn*, a straw mat or mattress. Its meanings eventually extended to include dependence, according, carry on, continue, reason, and cause.

Combinations
三因	〔三因〕	*sān yīn*	three causes (of disease)
内因	〔内因〕	*nèi yīn*	internal causes
外因	〔外因〕	*wài yīn*	external causes

Stroke Sequence

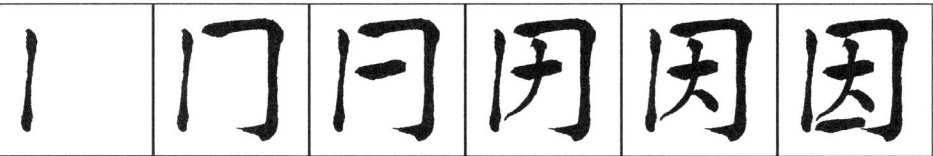

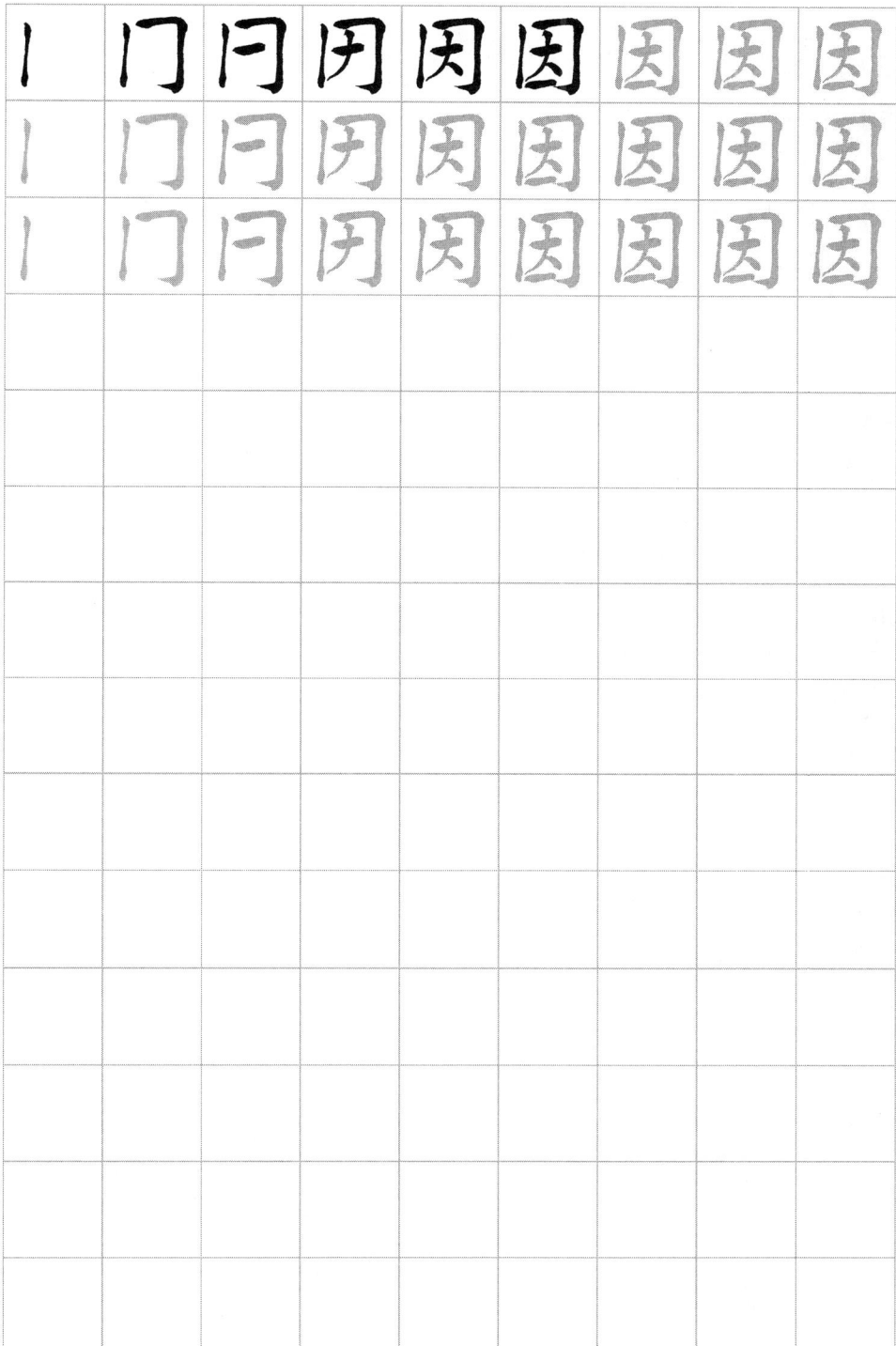

88. 邪〔邪〕 *xié* Evil

Equivalents
evil

Significs and Stroke Counts
simplified 阝 2 + 4; complex 邑（阝）7 (3) + 4

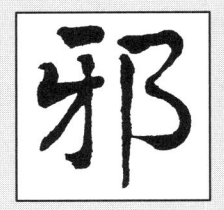

Character Composition

Signific-phonetic compound. On the right is the signific 阝 (邑 *yì*, town); on the left is 牙 *yá*, the phonetic.

Explanation

The signific component 邑 *yì* is composed of surrounding walls 囗 *wéi* and 卩 *jié*, an official seal, i.e., the city, the state. When 邑 *yì* is used as a signific, it is written as 阝 and is always placed on the right side of the character (阝 on the left is a different signific). The component on the left is 牙 *yá*, the teeth, which is the phonetic component. When the character is pronounced *xié* it bears the meaning of "evil" or "not upright," but the derivation of this meaning is unclear. In Chinese medicine, it is used to refer to all pathological causes.

Note that in certain complex character dictionaries, this character is to be found under the 7-stroke signific 邑, yet that signific is drawn with 3 strokes.

Combinations

邪气	〔邪氣〕	*xié qì*	evil qi
阴邪	〔陰邪〕	*yīn xié*	yīn evil
阳邪	〔陽邪〕	*yáng xié*	yáng evil
肺邪	〔肺邪〕	*fèi xié*	lung evil
实邪	〔實邪〕	*shí xié*	repletion evil
八邪	〔八邪〕	*bā xié*	Eight Evils (point name)
上八邪	〔上八邪〕	*shàng bā xié*	Upper Eight Evils (set of points)

Stroke Sequence

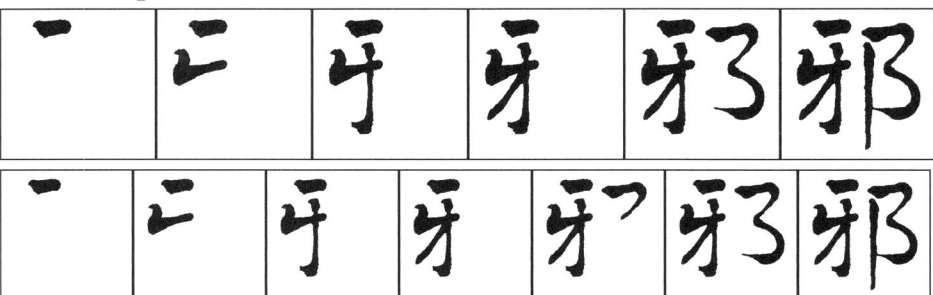

| 一 | 二 | 于 | 牙 | 牙阝 | 邪 | 邪 | 邪 | 邪 |

89. 淫〔淫〕 *yín* Excess

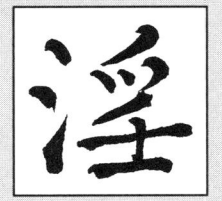

Equivalents

excess

Significs and Stroke Counts

simplified 氵 3 + 8; complex 水（氵） 4 (3) + 8

Character Composition

Signific-phonetic. On the left is the signific component 氵 *shuǐ*, water. On the right is the phonetic component *yín*.

Explanation

The phonetic component of this character may contribute to the meaning of the character. It depicts a downward facing hand, 爪 *zhuǎ*, seizing a part of a loom, 壬 *tíng*, to convey the meaning of encroaching. Thus the character 淫 *yín* means water seeping into something through seams or cracks (i.e., water encroaching). This meaning is reflected in the term 浸淫瘡 *jìn yín chuāng*, a "wet-spreading sore" or "seeping sore." In Chinese medicine, 淫 *yín* most commonly appears in the term 六淫 *liù yín*, the six excesses, which are the six environmental qì as forces that invade the body to cause disease.

It should be noted that outside medicine, 淫 *yín* is most commonly used in the sense of sexual licentiousness (淫穢 *yín huì*, obscene, salacious; 淫蕩 *yín dàng*, lascivious). In this meaning, it appears in the term 淫羊霍 *yín yáng huò*, epimedium, a medicinal used to treat impotence. The Chinese name of this medicinal means "lusty sheep plant."

Combinations

六淫　　〔六淫〕　　*liù yín*　　six excesses

Stroke Sequence

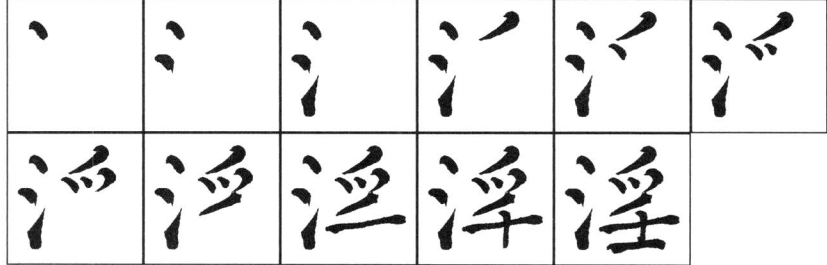

丶	丷	氵	汇	汀	汇	氾	泾	浮	淫
丶	丷	氵	汇	汀	汇	氾	泾	浮	淫
丶	丷	氵	汇	汀	汇	氾	泾	浮	淫

90. 风〔風〕 *fēng* Wind

Equivalents
wind

Significs and Stroke Counts
simplified 风 4; complex 風 9

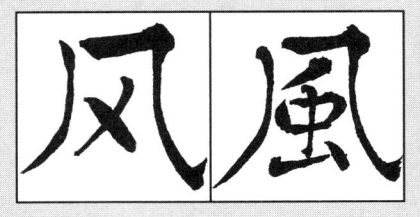

Character Composition

Associative compound. This character is composed of 凡 *fán,* which is also the phonetic element, and 虫 *chóng*, bugs or insects, which are said to breed when the wind blows.

Explanation

In lesser seal script, this character represented insects 虫 *chóng* that are borne on the wind. As the wind of spring brings insects to life, the association of wind with spring in the five phases is perhaps reflected in this character. The interior component is 虫 *chóng*, insects; the external component is 凡 *fán*, an early pictograph of an encompassing square that was often used in characters to symbolize the change associated with natural phenomena. Here it also serves a phonetic function.

Combinations

风邪	〔風邪〕	*fēng xié*	wind evil
中风	〔中風〕	*zhòng fēng*	wind strike
八风	〔八風〕	*bā fēng*	Eight Winds (set of points)
上八风	〔上八風〕	*shàng bā fēng*	Upper Eight Winds (set of points)

Stroke Sequence

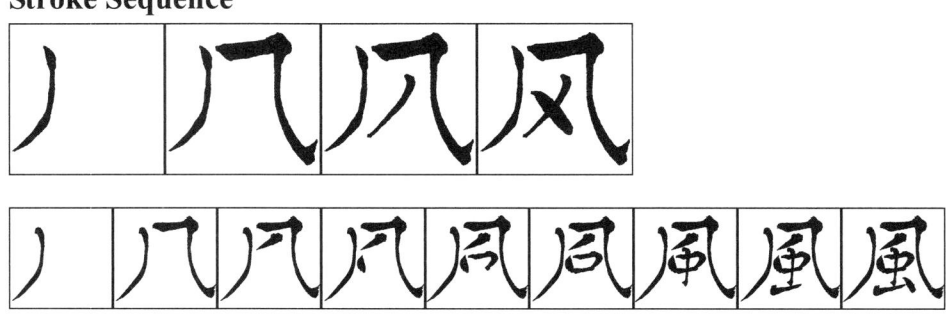

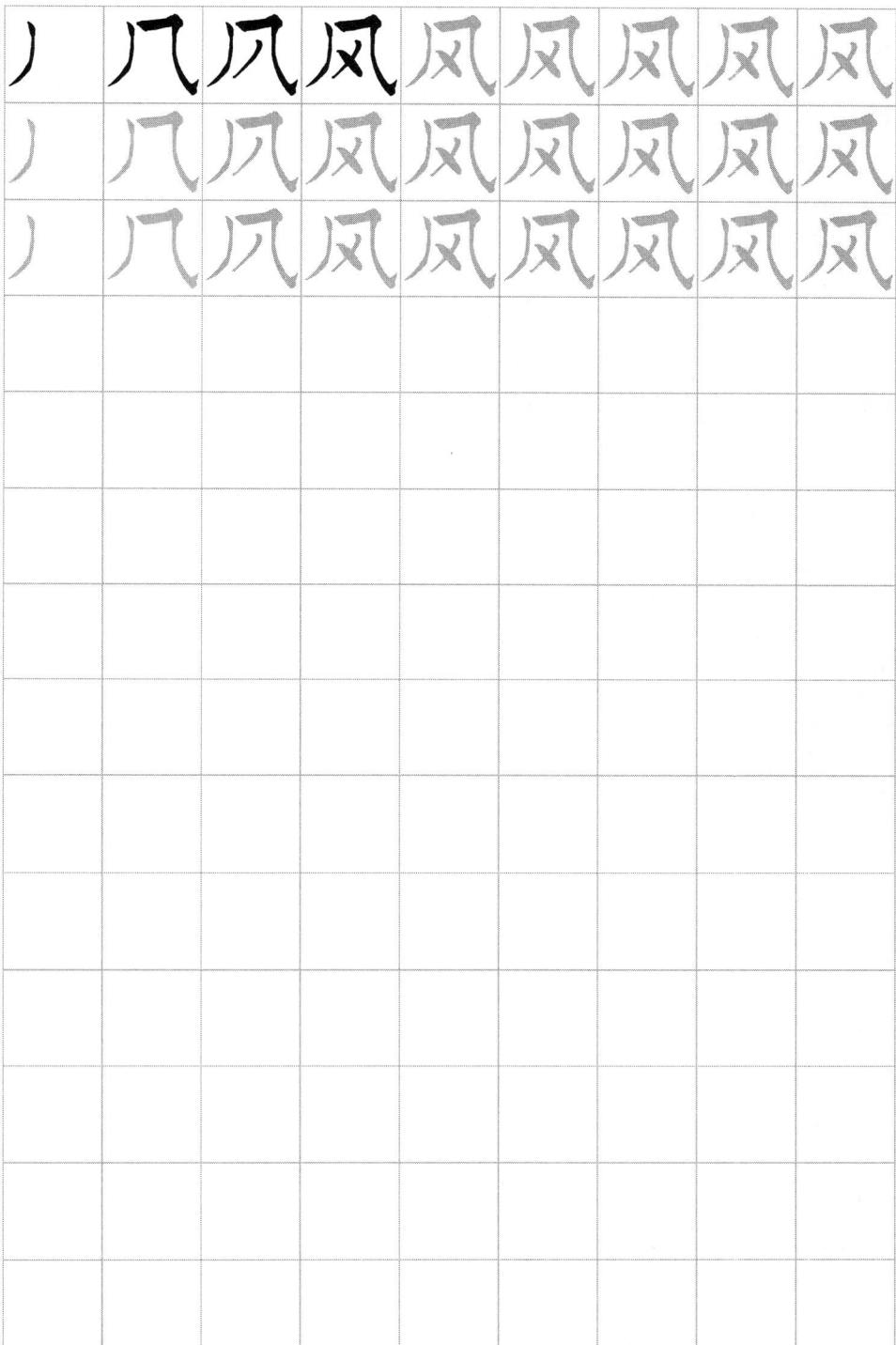

91. 寒〔寒〕 *hán* Cold

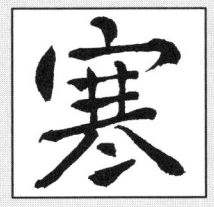

Equivalents

cold

Significs and Stroke Counts

simplified 宀 3 + 9; complex 宀 3 + 9

  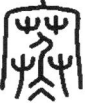

Character Composition

Ideograph. The character is composed of 宀 *mián*, "house" or "roof." Under the roof is the contracted form of the character 艸 *mǎng*, meaning an abundance of grasses. On the bottom is 仌 *bīng*, the ancient form of ice.

Explanation

The bronze inscriptions of the character depicts a person surrounded by a heap of thatch trying to stay warm under the roof. There are two lines under the man's feet as a symbol of ice. These two lines were simplified into two dots in later forms. Hence the original meaning of 寒 *hán* is cold. Coldness can produce shivering. By analogy, its extended meaning is fear, fearful trembling.

Combinations

寒邪	〔寒邪〕	*hán xié*	cold evil
邪寒	〔邪寒〕	*xié hán*	evil cold
风寒	〔風寒〕	*fēng hán*	wind-cold
中寒	〔中寒〕	*zhōng hán*	center cold
中寒	〔中寒〕	*zhòng hán*	cold strike
胃气虚寒	〔胃氣虛寒〕	*wèi qì xū hán*	stomach qì vacuity cold
大肠虚寒	〔大肠虛寒〕	*dà cháng xū hán*	large intestinal vacuity cold

Stroke Sequence

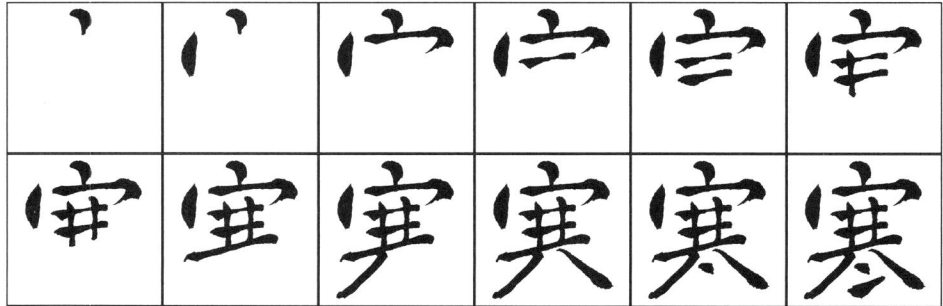

丶	宀	宀	宀	宁	宇	宙	宝	寅	寒	寒
丶	宀	宀	宀	宁	宇	宙	宝	寅	寒	寒
丶	宀	宀	宀	宁	宇	宙	宝	寅	寒	寒

92. 暑〔暑〕 *shǔ* Summerheat

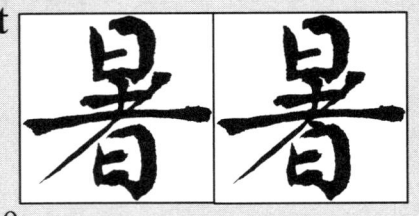

Equivalents
  summerheat

Significs and Stroke Counts
  simplified 日 4 + 8; complex 日 4 + 9

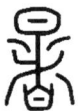

Character Composition
Signific-phonetic compound. On top is the signific component 日 *rì*, the sun. On the bottom is the phonetic component 者 *zhě*.

Explanation
This is another character for which the phonetic simply acts as a phonetic. Note that the complex character is only slightly different from the simplified, the difference being a single stroke.

Combinations

中暑	〔中暑〕	*zhòng shǔ*	summerheat strike
暑热	〔暑熱〕	*shǔ rè*	summerheat-heat
阳暑	〔陽暑〕	*yáng shǔ*	yáng summerheat
阴暑	〔陰暑〕	*yīn shǔ*	yīn summerheat
清暑热	〔清暑熱〕	*qīng shǔ rè*	clear summerheat-heat

Stroke Sequence

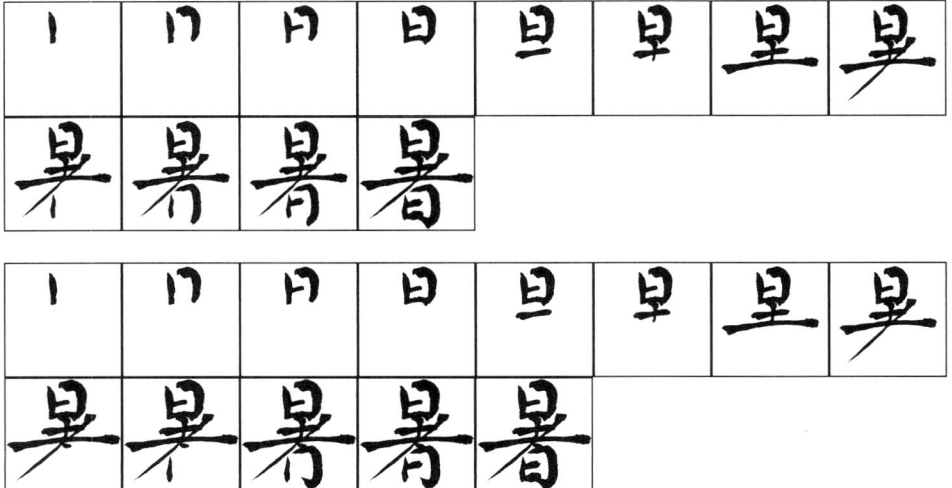

丿	冂	冃	日	旦	早	星	昇	昇	暑	暑	暑
丿	冂	冃	日	旦	早	星	昇	昇	暑	暑	暑
丿	冂	冃	日	旦	早	星	昇	昇	暑	暑	暑

93. 湿〔濕〕shī Dampness

Equivalents
  dampness

Significs and Stroke Counts
  simplified 氵 3 + 9; complex 水（氵）4 (3) + 14

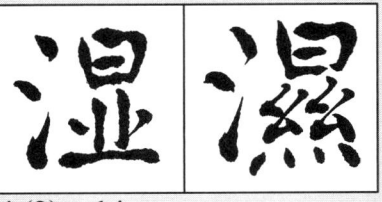

Character Composition

Signific-phonetic. On the left is the signific component 氵 *shuǐ,* water; on the right is the phonetic component 显 *xiǎn.*

Explanation

On the left is the signific component 氵 *shuǐ,* water. The phonetic component on the right is composed of 日 *rì,* the sun, on top and 絲 *sī,* silk, below.

There is another form of the complex character, 溼, which is now only seen in older texts.

Combinations

暑湿	〔暑濕〕	*shǔ shī*	summerheat-damp
寒湿	〔寒濕〕	*hán shī*	cold-damp
风寒湿	〔風寒濕〕	*fēng hán shī*	wind-cold-damp
风湿	〔風濕〕	*fēng shī*	wind-damp

Stroke Sequence

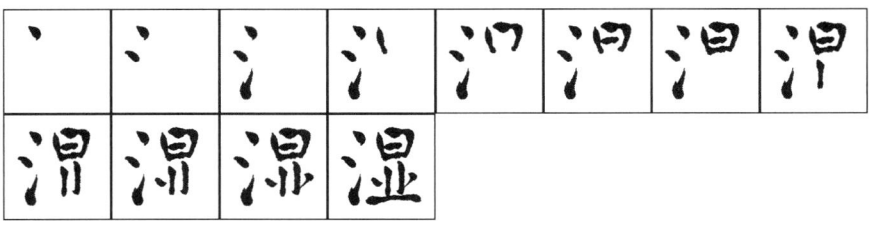

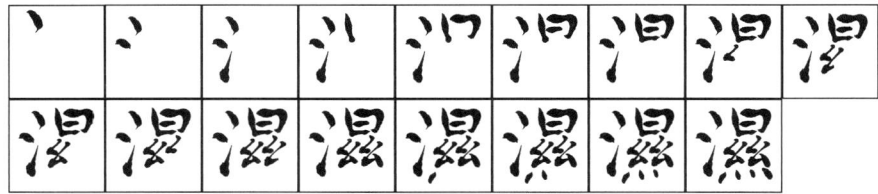

94. 燥 〔燥〕 *zào* **Dryness**

Equivalents

dry, dryness

Significs and Stroke Counts

simplified 火 4 + 13; complex 火 4 + 13

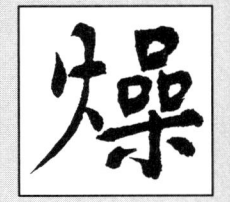

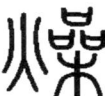

Character Composition

Signific-phonetic compound. On the left is the fire signific 火 *huǒ*; on the right the phonetic 喿 *zào*.

Explanation

The phonetic component on the right is composed of 品 *pǐn*, meaning a group of mouths, to taste, or a collection of small objects, on top of 木 *mù*, wood, tree. It is not clear how this association of components came to mean "dry."

Combinations

风燥	〔風燥〕	*fēng zào*	wind-dryness
肺燥	〔肺燥〕	*fèi zào*	lung dryness
鼻燥	〔鼻燥〕	*bí zào*	dry nose
口燥	〔口燥〕	*kǒu zào*	dry mouth
燥火	〔燥火〕	*zào huǒ*	dryness-fire

Stroke Sequence

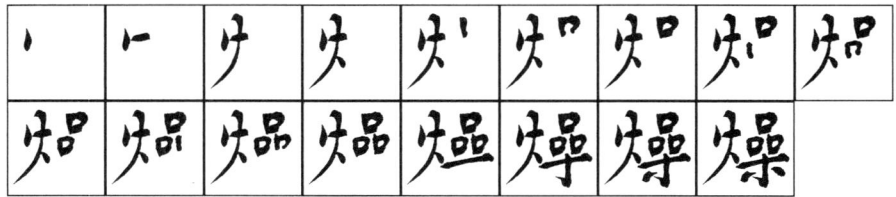

丶	一	ナ	大	大丶	大丷	大口	火口	炉	炉
焎	焔	焔	煙	煜	燥	燥	燥	燥	燥

95. 热〔熱〕 *rè* Heat

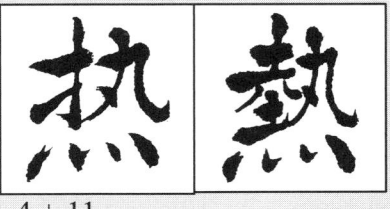

Equivalents
  heat

Significs and Stroke Counts
  simplified 灬 4 + 6; complex 火（灬）4 + 11

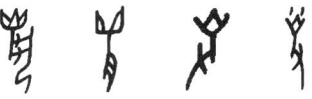

Character Composition

Associative compound. On top is the phonetic component 埶 *yì*, to hold. On the bottom is fire, 火(灬) *huǒ*.

Explanation

The top component is composed of 坴 *lù* on the left, meaning a large clod of dirt, and 丮 *jì* on the right, meaning a hand holding an object, or to hold. The oracle-bone form of the character indeed depicts a person holding a burning torch. Beginning with the lesser seal script, the fire signific was added to the bottom to signify the idea of heat, which is the basic meaning of this character.

Combinations

热邪	〔熱邪〕	*rè xié*	heat evil
风热	〔風熱〕	*fēng rè*	wind-heat
寒热	〔寒熱〕	*hán rè*	cold and heat
燥热	〔燥熱〕	*zào rè*	dryness heat
肺热	〔肺熱〕	*fèi rè*	lung heat
肝胆湿热	〔肝膽濕熱〕	*gān dǎn shī rè*	liver-gallbladder damp-heat
下焦湿热	〔下焦濕熱〕	*xià jiāo shī rè*	lower burner damp-heat
上寒下热	〔上寒下熱〕	*shàng hán xià rè*	upper-body cold, lower-body heat

Stroke Sequence

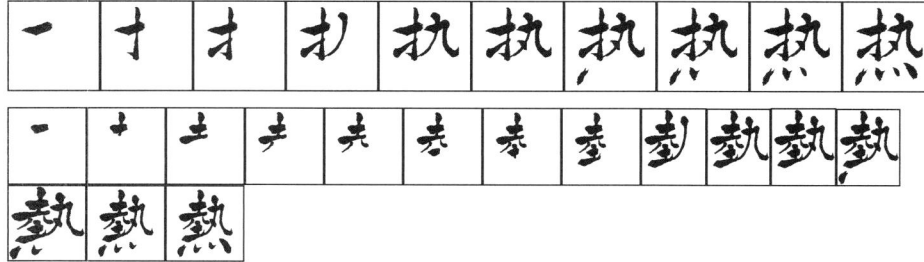

一	十	才	扎	执	执	执	热	热	热
一	十	才	扎	执	执	执	执	热	热
一	十	才	扎	执	执	执	执	热	热

96. 温〔溫〕 wēn Warm

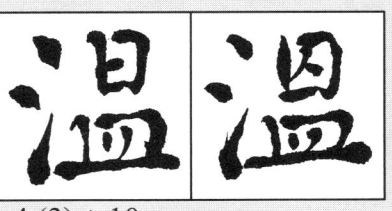

Equivalents
warm, warmth

Significs and Stroke Counts
simplified 氵 3 + 9; complex 水（氵） 4 (3) + 10

Character Composition
Signific-phonetic compound. On the left is the water signific 氵 shuǐ; on the right is the phonetic 昷 wēn.

Explanation
The phonetic may contribute to the meaning of this character. 昷 means benevolent, kind. In the complex character it is composed of an upper part 囚 qiú, which means a prisoner (and was changed to 日 rì in the simplified script), and a lower part 皿 mǐn, which means a bowl. It suggests giving a bowl of rice to a prisoner as an example of an act of kindness. The notion of warmth is represented by combining 昷 wēn with the water signific 氵 shuǐ, warmth being a water temperature that is gentle on the body.

Combinations

温邪	〔溫邪〕	wēn xié	warm evil
风温	〔風溫〕	fēng wēn	wind warmth
湿温	〔濕溫〕	shī wēn	damp warmth
温下	〔溫下〕	wēn xià	warm precipitation
温中	〔溫中〕	wēn zhōng	warm the center
暑温	〔暑溫〕	shǔ wēn	summerheat-warmth

Stroke Sequence

溫

97. 痰 〔痰〕 *tán* Phlegm

Equivalents
phlegm

Significs and Stroke Counts
simplified 疒 5 + 8; complex 疒 5 + 8

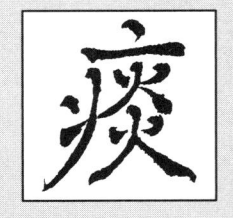

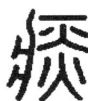

Character Composition

Signific-phonetic compound. The sickbed signific 疒 *nè* is combined with 炎 *yán*, the phonetic.

Explanation

The component 炎 *yán*, which means to flame, may also add to the meaning if it reflects an early conception of heat as a cause of phlegm.

The outer part is the signific component 疒 *nè*, to lie on a bed, that is extended to mean illness. Chinese characters formed with this component are virtually all related to illness or disease. The inner component is 炎 *yán*, flame. It is constructed by duplication of the character 火 *huǒ*, one on top of the other. These two components give rise to the idea of sickness erupting like flames, i.e., phlegm.

It is interesting to note that the English equivalent, phlegm, comes from the Greek *phlegein,* to burn.

Combinations

热痰	〔熱痰〕	*rè tán*	heat phlegm
寒痰	〔寒痰〕	*hán tán*	cold phlegm
燥痰	〔燥痰〕	*zào tán*	dryness phlegm
风痰	〔風痰〕	*fēng tán*	wind phlegm
痰涎	〔痰涎〕	*tán xián*	phlegm-drool

Stroke Sequence

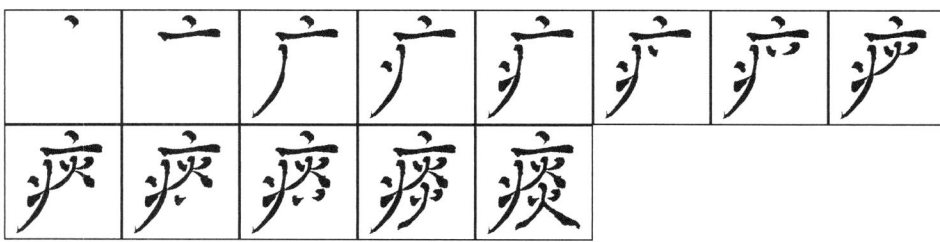

丶 亠 广 广 疒 疒 疒 疢 痰 痰 痰 痰
痰 痰 痰 痰 痰 痰 痰 痰

98. 饮〔飲〕yǐn Drink, Rheum

Equivalents

drink, rheum, fluid intake

Significs and Stroke Counts

simplified 饣 3 + 4; complex 食 9 (8) + 4

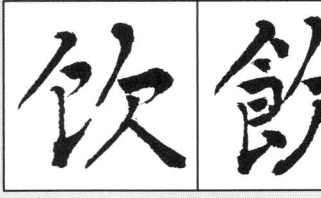

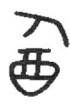 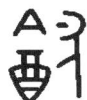 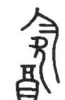 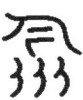 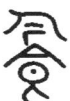 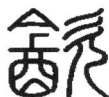

Character Composition

Associative compound. On the left is 食 *shí*, which represents a food jar; on the right is 欠 *qiàn*, meaning releasing of breath.

Explanation

In the bronze inscriptions the character depicts a man bending over a wine jar. Variants of the bronze-inscription character depict a man holding the wine jar in his arms with his tongue pointing to it. Its original meaning is to drink wine. However, its meaning was extended to include drinking in general as well as the drink, i.e., liquid, and, in medical terms, rheum.

Note that the signific is sometimes drawn with 8 strokes, as shown here, and sometimes drawn with 9 strokes, as demonstrated in the following character.

Combinations

痰饮	〔痰飲〕	*tán yǐn*	phlegm-rheum
寒饮	〔寒飲〕	*hán yǐn*	cold rheum
水饮	〔水飲〕	*shuǐ yǐn*	water-rheum
四饮	〔四飲〕	*sì yǐn*	the four rheums
饮邪	〔飲邪〕	*yǐn xié*	rheum evil

Stroke Sequence

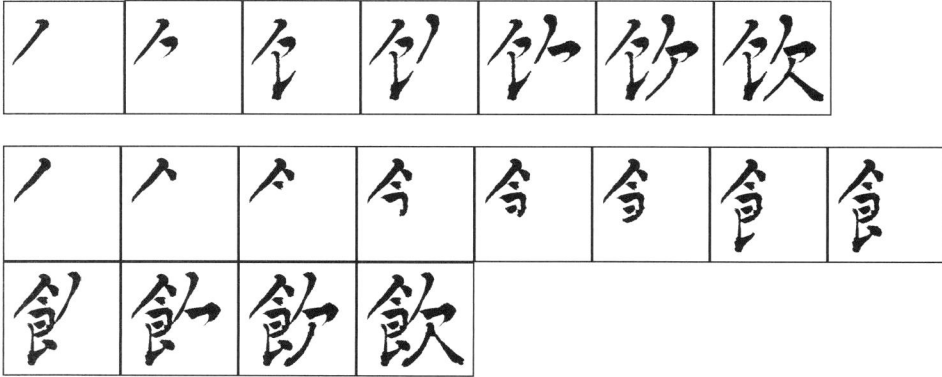

饮

99. 食〔食〕 *shí* Eat, Food

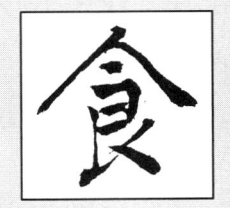

Equivalents

eat, food, diet, suckle, consume, meal

Significs and Stroke Counts

simplified 食 9; complex 食 9

  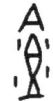   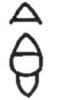

Character Composition

A pictograph representing a food jar.

Explanation

The ancient form of the character depicts a food jar with rice inside. Some interpretations suggest that the upper part of the character depicts a mouth that is upside-down and open, indicating the act of eating. Thus the meaning of the character: food, eating.

Combinations

饮食	〔飲食〕	*yǐn shí*	food and drink
食痰	〔食痰〕	*shí tán*	food-phlegm
痰食	〔痰食〕	*tán shí*	phlegm-food
生食	〔生食〕	*shēng shí*	eat raw
食中	〔食中〕	*shí zhòng*	food stroke

Stroke Sequence

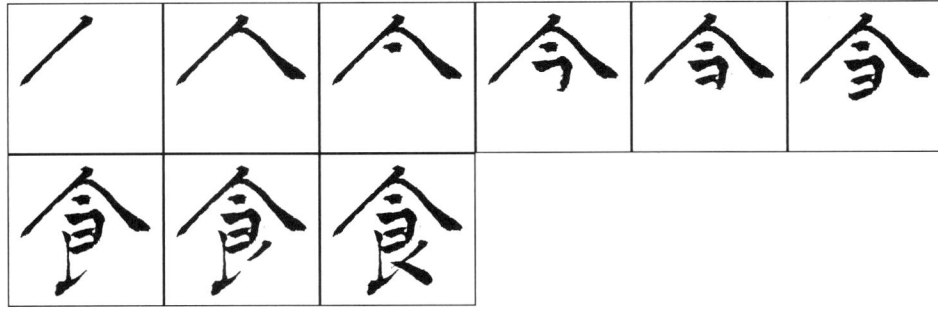

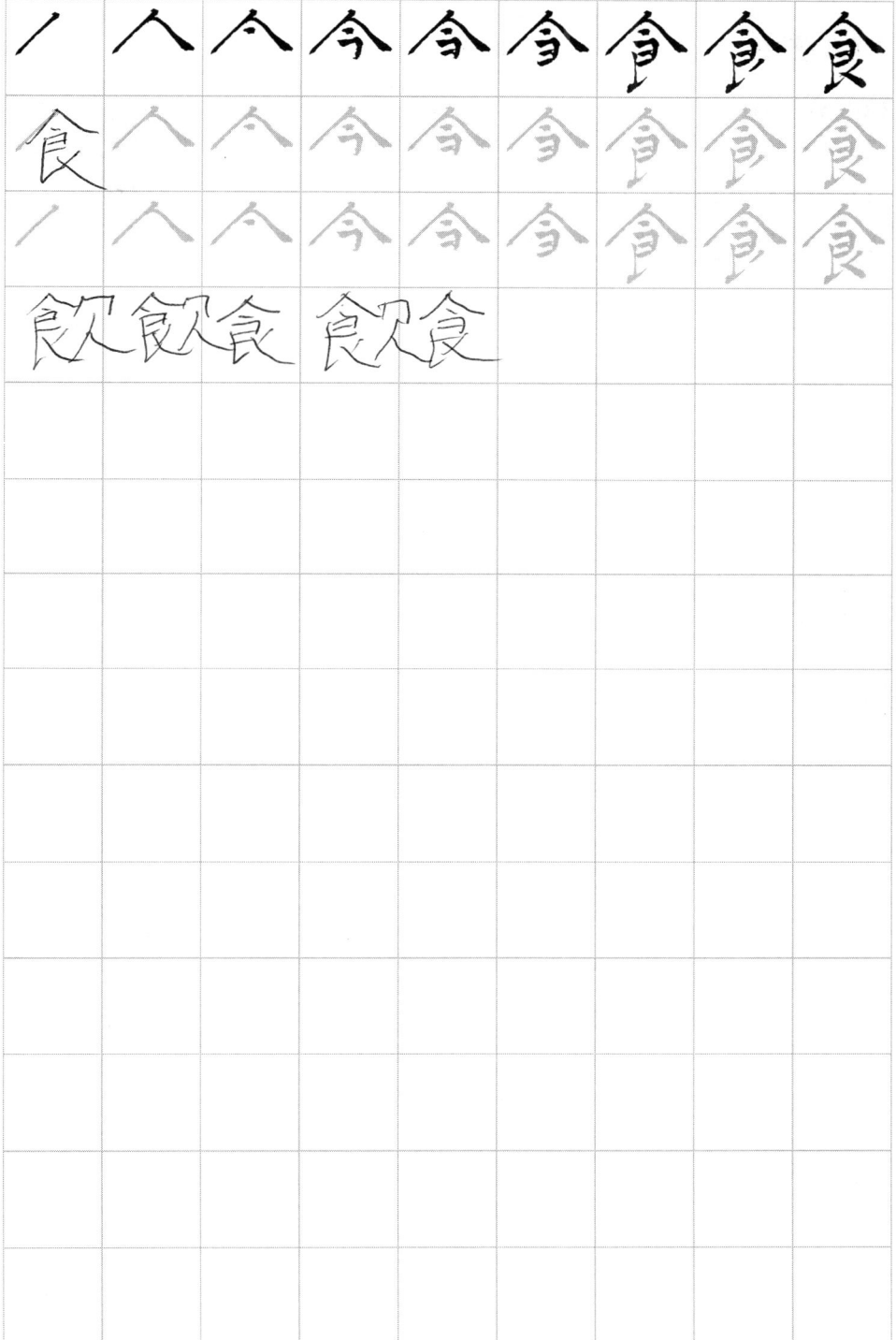

100. 瘀 〔瘀〕 *yū* Stasis

Equivalents
stasis

Significs and Stroke Counts
simplified 疒 5 + 8; complex 疒 5 + 8

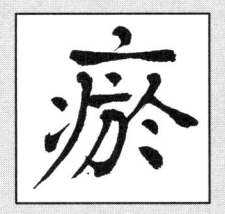

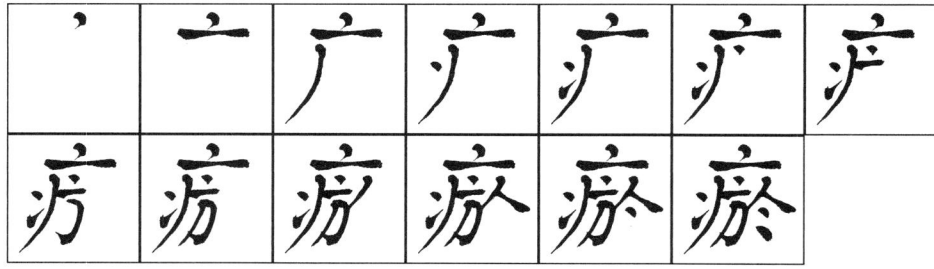

Character Composition

Signific-phonetic compound. The illness signific 疒 *nè* with 於 *yū* as a phonetic.

Explanation

Sometimes it is thought the phonetic component 於 *yú* contributes to the meaning of the character. 於 may represent 淤 *yū*, silt, sludge, in which case 瘀 *yū* would mean a pathological phenomenon analogous to silting.

Combinations

瘀血	〔瘀血〕	*yū xuè*	static blood
血瘀	〔血瘀〕	*xuè yū*	blood stasis

Stroke Sequence

、 亠 广 疒 疒 疒 疒 疖 疖 疖 瘀 瘀 瘀

肝〔肝〕*gān* Liver

Bibliography

Coulmas F (1989) *Writing Systems of the World.* Oxford: Blackwell.

Creel H (1939) *Literary Chinese by the Inductive Method.* Chicago: University of Chicago Press.

Dawson R (1984) *A New Introduction to Classical Chinese.* Oxford: Oxford University Press.

Fazzioli E (1987) *Charactères chinois: du dessin à l'idée, 214 clés pour comprendre la Chine.* Paris: Flammarion.

Flaws B (1998) *Teach Yourself to Read Modern Medical Chinese: A Step-by-Step Workbook and Guide.* Boulder: Blue Poppy Press.

McNaughton W (1979) *Reading and Writing Chinese: A Guide to the Chinese System.* Tokyo and Rutland: Tuttle Language Library.

Norman J (1988) *Chinese.* Cambridge Language Surveys Series. Cambridge: Cambridge University Press.

Ramsey S R (1987) *Languages of China.* Princeton: Princeton University Press.

Wáng Hóngyuán (王宏源) (1994) *Aux sources de l'écriture chinoise.* Beijing: Sinolingua.

Wieger L (1965) *Chinese Characters: Their Origin, Etymology, History, Classification and Signification.* New York: Paragon Book Reprint Corp., Dover Publications, Inc.

Wilder G D and Ingram J H (1972) *Analysis of Chinese Characters.* Taipei: Ch'eng Wen Publishing Company.

高鴻縉 (1950, 9th edition 2000)《中国字例》. Táiběi 台北: Sān-Mín Book Company 三民书局.

汉语大字典编辑委员会 (1986) 《汉语大字典》. Sìchuān 四川, Húběi 湖北: Sìchuān Lexicographical Publishing 四川辞书出版社, Húběi Lexicographical Publishing 湖北辞书出版社.

胡双宝 (1998)《汉语 汉字 汉文化》. Běijīng 北京: Běijīng University Press 北京大学出版社.

刘志成 (1995) 《汉字与华夏文化》. Sìchuān 四川: Bā Shǔ Book Publishing 巴蜀书社。

罗秋昭《有趣的中国字》. Táiběi 台北: Wǔ-Nán Book Publishing 五南图书出板公司。

水野惠 (1984)《古汉字典》. Tokyo: Mitsumura Shuiko Shoin Publishing Co. Ltd. 株式会社光村推古书院。

王鼎吉(1996)《字的基本知识 60 题》. Běijīng 北京: China Peace Press 中国和平出版社。

王宏源 (2000)《字里乾坤》. Běijīng 北京: Sinolingua 华语教育出版社。

吴颐人 (1994)《常用汉字演变图说》. Shànghǎi 上海: Shànghǎi Bookstore Publishing House 上海书店出版社。

谢光辉 (2000)《汉字字源字典》. Běijīng 北京: Běijīng University Press 北京大学出版社。

Pīnyīn Index

Numbering refers to character numbers, not page numbers.

bā, eight 八, 11
bái, white 白, 80
bāo, envelop 包, 56
bí, nose 鼻, 71
biǎo, exterior 表, 21
cháng, intestine 肠, 50
chì, red 赤, 78
dà, large 大, 14
dǎn, gallbladder 胆, 51
dì, earth 地, 3
ěr, ear 耳, 72
èr, two 二, 5
fèi, lung 肺, 48
fēng, wind 风, 90
fǔ, bowel 腑, 44
gān, liver 肝, 45
gǔ, bone 骨, 64
guāng, bladder 胱, 54
hán, cold 寒, 91
hàn, sweat 汗, 83
hēi, black 黑, 81
huáng, yellow 黄, 79
huǒ, fire 火, 31
jī, flesh 肌, 61
jiāo, burner, scorch 焦, 55
jīn, metal 金, 33
jīn, liquid 津, 39
jīn, sinew 筋, 58
jīng, essence 精, 41
jīng, channel 经, 73
jiǔ, nine 九, 12
kāi, open 开, 66
kè, restrain 克, 36
kǒu, mouth 口, 70

lèi, tears 泪, 82
lǐ, interior 里, 22
liù, six 六, 9
luò, network vessel 络, 74
mài, vessel 脉, 59
máo, body hair 毛, 63
miàn, face 面, 75
mù, wood 木, 30
mù, eye 目, 68
nèi, internal 内, 19
páng, bladder 膀, 53
pí, spleen 脾, 47
pí, skin 皮, 62
qī, seven 七, 10
qì, qì 气, 37
qiào, orifice 窍, 65
qīng, clear 清, 23
qīng, green-blue 青, 77
rè, heat 热, 95
rén, human 人, 2
ròu, flesh 肉, 60
sān, three 三, 6
sè, color, complexion 色, 76
shàng, up 上, 17
shé, tongue 舌, 69
shén, spirit 神, 42
shèn, kidney 肾, 49
shēng, engender 生, 35
shī, dampness 湿, 93
shí, ten 十, 13
shí, repletion 实, 26
shí, food, eat 食, 00
shǔ, summerheat 暑, 92

shuǐ, water 水, 34
sì, four 四, 7
tán, phlegm 痰, 97
tì, snivel 涕, 85
tiān, heaven 天, 1
tǔ, earth 土, 32
tuò, spittle 唾, 86
wài, external 外, 20
wèi, stomach 胃, 52
wēn, warmth 温, 96
wǔ, five 五, 8
xià, down 下, 18
xián, drool 涎, 84
xiǎo, small 小, 15
xié, evil 邪, 88
xīn, heart 心, 46
xíng, move; phase 行, 29
xū, vacuity 虚, 25
xuè, blood 血, 38
yáng, yáng 阳, 28
yè, humor 液, 40
yī, one 一, 4
yīn, yīn 阴, 27
yīn, cause 因, 87
yín, excess 淫, 89
yǐn, drink; rheum 饮, 98
yū, stasis 瘀, 100
yú, at 于, 67
zàng, viscus 脏, 43
zào, dryness 燥, 94
zhōng, center 中, 16
zhǔ, govern 主, 57
zhuó, turbid 浊, 24

English Index

Numbering refers to character numbers, not page numbers.

black, *hēi* 黑, 81
bladder, *páng* 膀, 53
bladder, *guāng* 胱, 54
blood, *xuè* 血, 38
body hair, *máo* 毛, 63
bone, *gǔ* 骨, 64
bowel, *fǔ* 腑, 44
burner, scorch, *jiāo* 焦, 55
cause, *yīn* 因, 87
center, *zhōng* 中, 16
channel, *jīng* 经, 73
clear, *qīng* 清, 23
cold, *hán* 寒, 91
color, complexion, *sè* 色, 76
dampness, *shī* 湿, 93
down, *xià* 下, 18
drink; rheum, *yǐn* 饮, 98
drool, *xián* 涎, 84
dryness, *zào* 燥, 94
ear, *ěr* 耳, 72
earth, *dì* 地, 3
earth, *tǔ* 土, 32
eight, *bā* 八, 11
engender, *shēng* 生, 35
envelop, *bāo* 包, 56
essence, *jīng* 精, 41
evil, *xié* 邪, 88
excess, *yín* 淫, 89
exterior, *biǎo* 表, 21
external, *wài* 外, 20
eye, *mù* 目, 68
face, *miàn* 面, 75

fire, *huǒ* 火, 31
five, *wǔ* 五, 8
flesh, *ròu* 肉, 60
flesh, *jī* 肌, 61
food, eat, *shí* 食, 99
four, *sì* 四, 7
gallbladder, *dǎn* 胆, 51
govern, *zhǔ* 主, 57
green-blue, *qīng* 青, 77
heart, *xīn* 心, 46
heat, *rè* 热, 95
heaven, *tiān* 天, 1
human, *rén* 人, 2
humor, *yè* 液, 40
interior, *lǐ* 里, 22
internal, *nèi* 内, 19
intestine, *cháng* 肠, 50
kidney, *shèn* 肾, 49
large, *dà* 大, 14
liquid, *jīn* 津, 39
liver, *gān* 肝, 45
lung, *fèi* 肺, 48
metal, *jīn* 金, 33
mouth, *kǒu* 口, 70
move; phase, *xíng* 行, 29
network vessel, *luò* 络, 74
nine, *jiǔ* 九, 12
nose, *bí* 鼻, 71
one, *yī* 一, 4
open, *kāi* 开, 66
orifice, *qiào* 窍, 65
phlegm, *tán* 痰, 97
qì, *qì* 气, 37
red, *chì* 赤, 78

repletion, *shí* 实, 26
restrain, *kè* 克, 36
seven, *qī* 七, 10
sinew, *jīn* 筋, 58
six, *liù* 六, 9
skin, *pí* 皮, 62
small, *xiǎo* 小, 15
snivel, *tì* 涕, 85
spirit, *shén* 神, 42
spittle, *tuò* 唾, 86
spleen, *pí* 脾, 47
stasis, *yū* 瘀, 100
stomach, *wèi* 胃, 52
summerheat, *shǔ* 暑, 92
sweat, *hàn* 汗, 83
tears, *lèi* 泪, 82
ten, *shí* 十, 13
three, *sān* 三, 6
tongue, *shé* 舌, 69
turbid, *zhuó* 浊, 24
two, *èr* 二, 5
up, *shàng* 上, 17
vacuity, *xū* 虚, 25
vessel, *mài* 脉, 59
viscus, *zàng* 脏, 43
warmth, *wēn* 温, 96
water, *shuǐ* 水, 34
white, *bái* 白, 80
wind, *fēng* 风, 90
wood, *mù* 木, 30
yáng, *yáng* 阳, 28
yellow, *huáng* 黄, 79
yīn, *yīn* 阴, 27

Character Stroke Index

Numbering refers to character numbers, not page numbers.

1 Stroke
一 *yī*, one, 4

2 Strokes
七 *qī*, seven, 10
九 *jiǔ*, nine, 12
二 *èr*, two, 5
人 *rén*, human, 2
八 *bā*, eight, 11
十 *shí*, ten, 13

3 Strokes
三 *sān*, three, 6
上 *shàng*, up, 17
下 *xià*, down, 18
于 *yú*, at, 67
口 *kǒu*, mouth, 70
土 *tǔ*, earth, 32
大 *dà*, large, 14
小 *xiǎo*, small, 15

4 Strokes
中 *zhōng*, center, 16
五 *wǔ*, five, 8
六 *liù*, six, 9
内 *nèi*, internal, 19
天 *tiān*, heaven, 1
开 *kāi*, open, 66
心 *xīn*, heart, 46
木 *mù*, wood, 30
毛 *máo*, body hair, 63
气 *qì*, qì, 37
水 *shuǐ*, water, 34
火 *huǒ*, fire, 31
风 *fēng*, wind, 90

5 Strokes
主 *zhǔ*, govern, 57
包 *bāo*, envelop, 56
四 *sì*, four, 7
外 *wài*, external, 20
生 *shēng*, engender, 35

白 *bái*, white, 80
皮 *pí*, skin, 62
目 *mù*, eye, 68

6 Strokes
因 *yīn*, cause, 87
地 *dì*, earth, 3
汗 *hàn*, sweat, 83
耳 *ěr*, ear, 72
肉 *ròu*, flesh, 60
肌 *jī*, flesh, 61
舌 *shé*, tongue, 69
色 *sè*, color, complexion, 76
血 *xuè*, blood, 38
行 *xíng*, move; phase, 29
邪 *xié*, evil, 88
阳 *yáng*, yáng, 28
阴 *yīn*, yīn, 27

7 Strokes
克 *kè*, restrain, 36
肝 *gān*, liver, 45
肠 *cháng*, intestine, 50
赤 *chì*, red, 78
里 *lǐ*, interior, 22
饮 *yǐn*, drink; rheum, 98

8 Strokes
实 *shí*, repletion, 26
泪 *lèi*, tears, 82
经 *jīng*, channel, 73
肺 *fèi*, lung, 48
肾 *shèn*, kidney, 49
表 *biǎo*, exterior, 21
金 *jīn*, metal, 33
青 *qīng*, green-blue, 77

9 Strokes
津 *jīn*, liquid, 39
浊 *zhuó*, turbid, 24
涎 *xián*, drool, 84
神 *shén*, spirit, 42

络 *luò*, network vessel, 74
胃 *wèi*, stomach, 52
胆 *dǎn*, gallbladder, 51
脉 *mài*, vessel, 59
面 *miàn*, face, 75
食 *shí*, food, eat, 99
骨 *gǔ*, bone, 64

10 Strokes
涕 *tì*, snivel, 85
热 *rè*, heat, 95
窍 *qiào*, orifice, 65
胱 *guāng*, bladder, 54
脏 *zàng*, viscus, 43

11 Strokes
唾 *tuò*, spittle, 86
液 *yè*, humor, 40
淫 *yín*, excess, 89
清 *qīng*, clear, 23
虚 *xū*, vacuity, 25
黄 *huáng*, yellow, 79

12 Strokes
寒 *hán*, cold, 91
暑 *shǔ*, summerheat, 92
温 *wēn*, warmth, 96
湿 *shī*, dampness, 93
焦 *jiāo*, burner, scorch, 55
筋 *jīn*, sinew, 58
脾 *pí*, spleen, 47
腑 *fǔ*, bowel, 44
黑 *hēi*, black, 81

13 Strokes
痰 *tán*, phlegm, 97
瘀 *yū*, stasis, 100
精 *jīng*, essence, 41
膀 *páng*, bladder, 53
鼻 *bí*, nose, 71
燥 *zào*, dryness

CHINESE MEDICINE LANGUAGE SERIES

These works provide an ideal resource for those engaged in the study of Chinese medical language by facilitating acquisition of the root vocabulary and the conceptual context of Chinese medicine.

Each volume in an overall series of five books introduces 100 characters that are common to the specific vocabulary. Simplified and complex forms, significs and stroke counts, commonly used equivalents, character composition, explanation of meaning, and examples of character combinations are included. The stroke sequence showing how to write the character is presented, and space for students to practice writing the characters is provided. Additionally there is an appendix that contains a systematic list of all the characters introduced in previous volumes. You can use this for review purposes. These books will help you achieve both competence and mastery in medical language understanding and acquisition.

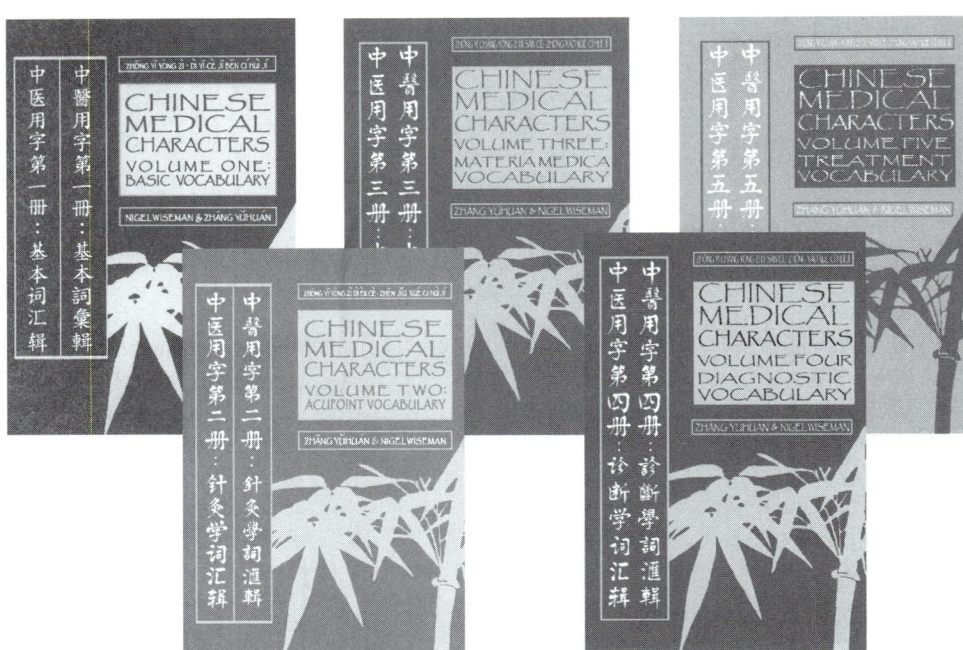

Paradigm Publications ~ Taos NM
www.paradigm-pubs.com
distributed by Redwing Book Company, www.redwingbooks.com